## Praise for *Natural Remedies*

"Laura is a wealth of knowledge and e̷____ _____ ____ __ essential oils. She has designed so many amazing recipes and ways to use essential oils, and she is so inspiring when it comes to living a more natural lifestyle!"

—Marissa Tolsma, founder of the blog *Bumblebee Apothecary*

"You'll find Laura's approach to natural living to be encouraging, nonintimidating, and most of all—inspirational! As a busy mom to five kiddos, this book feels like everything I need to transform our home into a more healthy environment and has given me so many ideas for swapping out the remainder of our commercial products for ones I feel more confident using to clean our home and apply to our bodies. Laura makes it fun, easy, and lights a fire in me to keep going!"

—Cami Graham, founder of the blog *Tidbits* and author of *Master the Electric Pressure Cooker*

"Laura is my go-to source for all things essential oils … I can always count on her for a natural remedy that's simple, and most importantly, effective!"

—Andrea, founder of the blog *Pine and Prospect Home*

"Laura is an authority on using essential oils in every part of your life— from food, to beauty products, to homemade cleaners. *A Mom's Guide to a Healthy Home* gives us practical, eco-conscious advice and tested recipes to help us create a safer home. This book is a keeper!"

—Pam Farley, founder of the blog *Brown Thumb Mama* and author of *Complete Essential Oil Diffuser Recipes*

# NATURAL REMEDIES *for* YOUR HOME & HEALTH

# NATURAL REMEDIES *for* YOUR HOME & HEALTH

DIY Essential Oil Recipes for Cleaning,
Beauty, and Wellness

LAURA ASCHER

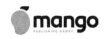

mango
PUBLISHING GROUP

CORAL GABLES

Cover Design: Elina Diaz
Cover Photo/illustration: Laura Ascher
Layout & Design: Elina Diaz

For permission requests, please contact the publisher at:
Mango Publishing Group
2850 S Douglas Road, 2nd Floor
Coral Gables, FL 33134 USA
info@mango.bz

For special orders, quantity sales, course adoptions and corporate sales, please email the publisher at sales@mango.bz. For trade and wholesale sales, please contact Ingram Publisher Services at customer.service@ingramcontent.com or +1.800.509.4887.

Natural Remedies for Your Home & Health: DIY Essential Oil Recipes for Cleaning, Beauty, and Wellness

Library of Congress Cataloging-in-Publication number: 2021931799
ISBN: (print) 978-1-64250-548-1, (ebook) 978-1-64250-549-8
BISAC category code: HEA029000—HEALTH & FITNESS / Aromatherapy

Printed in the United States of America

To my husband, Nathan. Without his help, this book would not be published. He supports all of my business endeavors and willingly helped me with the kids and household chores so I could write and photograph this book.

# Table of Contents

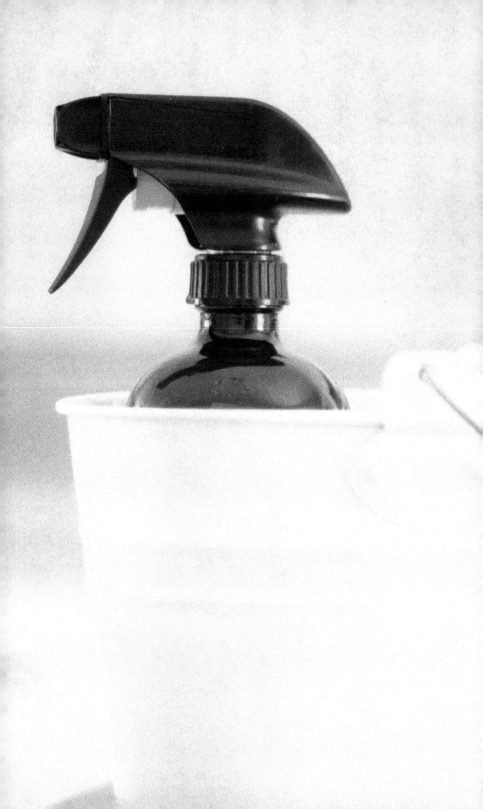

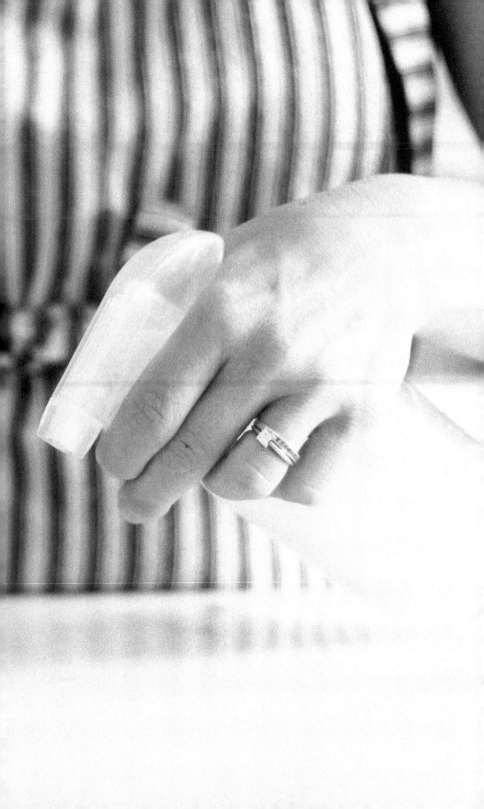

# Foreword

For as long as I can remember, my sister Laura has loved babies more than anyone I've ever known. With our dad being the tenth child of fourteen, our family Christmas parties always had at least one small cousin for Laura to tote around between opening presents and eating pumpkin pie. When our mom finally had another little girl, six years after her, Laura faked being sick from school so she could stay home with the chubby newborn.

After years of experience nannying multiple littles in her teens and early twenties, I just knew Laura would be fully prepared to assume her role as a mother just under ten months into marriage. But when she held her tiny Caroline in her arms for the first time, she started researching and questioning everything. "What's in this highly scented baby shampoo?" "What if the baby gets into the toxic cleaners under the sink?" Her fiercely protective mothering instincts drove her to create a more natural home that would be safe for her precious little family. Through trial, error, research, and experience, Laura has created a natural solution for everything from face serums to dish soap.

I have always admired Laura for her dedication to keeping her family healthy, often bypassing convenience to stand by her conviction to avoid chemical-laden commercial goods.

Five kids later, Laura is every bit as passionate and infinitely more knowledgeable about creating a healthy home, whether you live in a tiny apartment or sprawling farmhouse. In our family and friend group, she is the go-to gal for all things essential oils and natural living. I'm sure this book is partially in response to the thousands of questions she gets every year, "Hey Laura, what oil should I use if I have a poison ivy rash on my arm?" "What do you use for a body wash that doesn't contain sodium laureth sulfate?"

Now her friends, family, and the world can access her wealth of knowledge between the pages of this book. Whether you are a new parent, just graduated and moved into your first apartment, or simply want a cleaner, toxin-free lifestyle, you will find something in this book for you! I know I'll keep it handy to reference next time I pull out my phone to text her, "What oil can I use to get this red sharpie off the floor?!" With this beautiful guide, you, too, will have a direct line to Laura's knowledge to create your own natural, toxin-free home.

**Lisa Bass**
Founder of the blog *Farmhouse on Boone*
and author of *Simple Farmhouse Life*

# My Story

My name is Laura, and I am the face behind the blog and YouTube channel *Our Oily House*. I am a wife and a mother of five, so, needless to say, things can get pretty busy around here. I grew up in the Midwest on a large elk farm with four hundred acres to explore. As one of four girls, and have fond childhood memories of playing in the creek, jumping on hay bales, and helping my dad take care of all of the animals. We also had cattle, horses, dogs, and cats. Growing up surrounded by nature has shaped who I am and has made me want to provide as healthy and sustainable a life as possible for my own family (and hopefully help you on this path, too).

After high school, I went on to get my associate's degree and started nannying. I've always loved kids, and being a "mommy" for the day was just the job for me. I got married in 2012 to my husband Nathan, and we welcomed our first child into our family in 2013. A few short months after Caroline was born, I found out I was expecting our second child. At this time, I decided to step back from nannying and stay home with my kids. I have been a stay-at-home mom ever since and truly love it.

Soon after having my daughter is when natural remedies and essential oils entered my life. I loved the idea of having natural solutions on hand when my babies needed them, and I was eager to replace conventional products in my home with natural, homemade options. I was first introduced to essential oils when a friend invited me to an oil class and loved it so much that I bought my first set of oils that day! I started using my essential oils right away and quickly couldn't imagine life before them.

A couple of months after having my fourth baby, I decided to start my blog and YouTube channel. Friends and family had begun asking for my recommendations on natural remedies, and I wanted a place to compile

all of my research and recipes. I never imagined that my little hobby
would turn into a full-blown business that I loved. Sharing my recipes and
helping other people feel empowered to use essential oils for natural
solutions is my true passion.

My family of seven currently lives on a small, three-acre homestead, if
I can even call it that. We have chickens in our backyard and grow as
many vegetables as possible in our garden, just like when I grew up. We
have dreams of moving to a larger farm someday to be even more self-
sufficient, but we are content for now. I am passionate about feeding
my family wholesome meals and love to create new recipes. I spend a
lot of time in the kitchen, usually with a baby in tow and a toddler on the
counter. Most nights, we eat a home-cooked meal of grass-fed meat,
vegetables, and something fermented. We strive to live a simple life with
lots of time spent outside and family dinners every night. As this book is
in your hands, I'll bet you're interested in this kind of simpler, slower, and
more natural kind of life as well!

In this book, I share recipes to transform each room in your home into
a healthier place by filling it with more natural options. From cleaning
products to makeup and roller bottle blends, I hope this book inspires
you and that you find it helpful as you jump into using essential oils in
your home.

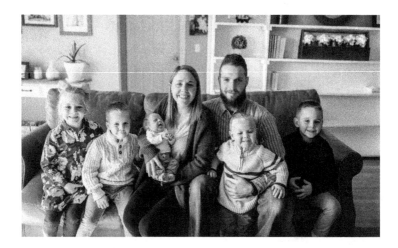

# Getting Started

I assume if you are still reading, you are ready to jump into revamping your living space to make it a safer place. Am I right?

I am so excited to take you through each room of your home and show you how to make it a healthier space with natural, homemade products.

Before we jump right in, let's discuss the supplies you will need. These tried-and-true materials and tips will make this whole process less stressful, and it's good to address some safety concerns before starting as well.

## What Will I Need?

Each recipe will have its own list of ingredients and instructions, but you will see that many recipes will call for similar things. (All of which are affordable and easy to find.) As we go through this journey together, you will learn I like to keep things easy, and I love recipes with minimal ingredients. If I ever see a recipe with a long list of ingredients, I find myself skipping over it. Who has the time for that, right? Like you, I am very busy and like to keep things simple for my sanity.

Some materials you will often find throughout this book include:

**BAKING SODA**: The first ingredient I reach for when I am creating a new cleaning product is baking soda. If you read the description on your average baking soda box, it will have a whole section about using it for cleaning and laundry. Baking soda is an effective odor remover and can leave your house smelling fresh and clean. It is a great natural cleaning agent and has been used for cleaning for many, many years. With its mild alkali properties, it can cause dirt, grime, and grease to dissolve quickly. Baking soda is effective for removing soap scum, hard water, and it also helps with whitening. In sum, a miracle product!

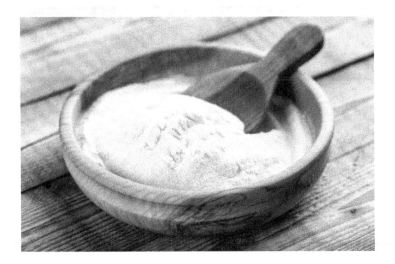

**WASHING SODA**: Washing soda is sodium carbonate that dissolves in water for washing and cleaning. It is a natural cleaner and can be used to soften water. Washing soda is also neutralizing and eliminates odors.

**VINEGAR:** Vinegar is great for cleaning because of its high acidity level. It can remove sticky buildup, dissolve soap scum, get rid of rings left by hard water, and cut grease. Vinegar can also kill salmonella and E.coli—two bacteria you don't want anywhere near your home.

**CASTILE SOAP:** OK, I might as well admit this now because you are going to find out soon enough: I am obsessed with castile soap. Castile soap is gentle, safe, and leaves surfaces squeaky clean. It is highly concentrated, making it cost-effective because you only need a little bit each time you clean, and each bottle will last you a long time. I prefer to use the unscented kind to use my essential oils to scent it the way I want.

**ESSENTIAL OILS:** You probably already assumed that essential oils would be a big part of this book, especially if you have checked out my blog or YouTube channel, *Our Oily House*. Throughout the book, you will find diffuser blends, roller bottle recipes, and lots of natural DIYs with essential oils. So stock up on your favorites!

**COCONUT OIL:** Coconut oil can be found in many skincare products for good reasons. It can protect the skin against anti-aging, dryness, imperfections, and even infections. Coconut oil is naturally anti-bacterial and anti-fungal, and it is moisturizing for the skin. It is primarily made up of nourishing fatty acids and is high in lauric acid. It contains vitamin E and several healthy fats that help to make skin smooth. When purchasing coconut oil, unrefined and organic is best, especially if you plan to use it in the kitchen. For skin and hair, expeller-pressed, fractionated, or other types of refined coconut oil will work.

**SHEA BUTTER:** I love the light earthy smell of shea butter. It goes perfectly in so many of my bath and beauty recipes. It has a high concentration of fatty acids and vitamins that are great for the skin. Using shea butter on your body can improve skin tone, moisturize, and soothe. Because it is so gentle, it is great for all skin types.

**COCOA BUTTER:** Cocoa butter is the fat that comes from cocoa beans, and it smells delicious, in my opinion. Cocoa butter naturally moisturizes the skin and heals dry, chapped skin. Fair warning, it smells like chocolate, and you may be tempted to eat your skincare products! (Don't worry, cocoa butter is edible and used to make delicate chocolates.)

**BEESWAX:** Beeswax is another one of those ingredients you will see a lot of, especially when it comes to skincare. With its antiviral, anti-inflammatory, and antibacterial properties, this ingredient is the best for damaged or dry skin. It forms a protective wall by sealing moisture in the skin without clogging up the pores.

**DOUBLE BOILER:** You will notice that a lot of the skincare recipes call for a double boiler. A double boiler ensures that the ingredients don't get burnt when you are melting them together. You can buy one pretty inexpensively at any box store or online. If you do not have one, you can make your own by placing a glass or stainless steel bowl inside a pot of boiling water.

## 4 Tips Before Diving In

1.  Take this one product at a time. Don't think you have to throw everything in your house away and make all the things overnight. This is a process, and slow is okay.

2.  Just jump right in! There is no reason to wait or overthink this. It is so much easier once you get started, so just start. Pick one recipe that calls to you, make it, use it, and move on to the next. The only way to discover which ones work the best for you is by trying them out!

3.  Label everything. Okay, I'll be the first to tell you that *you will forget* what is in the glass spray bottle with no label. I always think I'll remember or trust that the kids won't switch things up on me, but that isn't reality. It doesn't have to be fancy if you make your own, but label everything. **At the back of this book, I have included labels for all the recipes in this book that you can cut out and paste on your containers.** Thank me later!

4.  Store every product made with essential oils in glass, metal, or an HDPE plastic container, also known as plastic number 2. This is because essential oils can dissolve some plastics overtime. Store DIYs out of direct sunlight and in dark-colored glass to preserve the potency of the essential oils.

## Using Essential Oils Safely

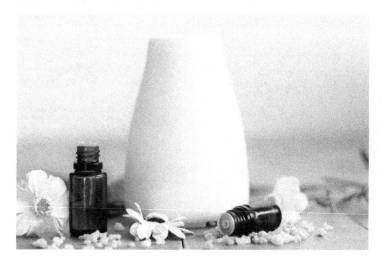

Essential oils are very potent and concentrated—a little goes a long way. When putting them into skincare products, be sure to dilute them properly and always test them on your foot or somewhere with less sensitive skin.

It is best to apply essential oils to the area of concern, down the spine, on pulse points, or the bottom of your feet. It is important to note that you should never put essential oils in your ears or eyes.

I love using essential oils on my kids and diffusing oils to help with sleep, mood, and so much more. It is important to remember to keep essential oils out of children's reach and only let them use them under adult supervision.

Now, who's ready to make some natural remedies?

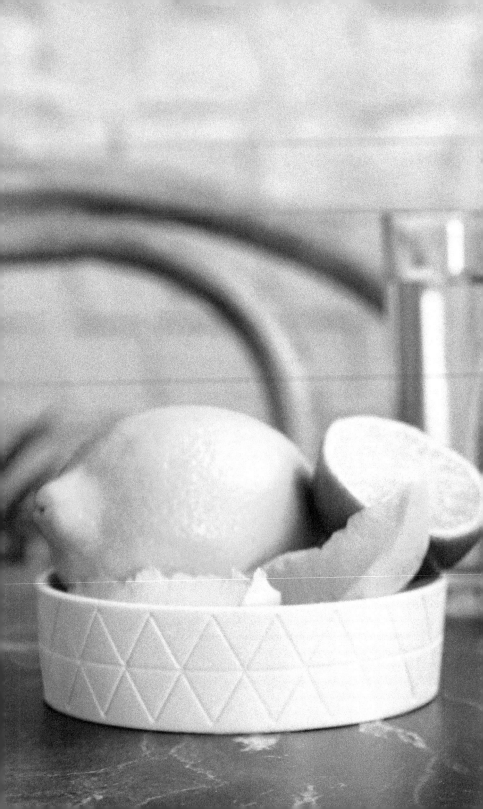

# CHAPTER ONE
# Natural Kitchen Remedies

As a wife and mother of five little ones, I spend a lot of time in the kitchen. As soon as one meal is done, it is time to start prepping for the next. Oh, and then there are the snacks! Feeding and cleaning up after my family can seem like a never-ending job.

Having natural cleaners and products in my kitchen is important to me for a couple of reasons. First off, I am picky with what my family eats, and I like to buy organic and fresh produce when I can. I would hate to ruin good food with chemical-filled cookware and cleaners. Second, I love to let my kids help in the kitchen. They are still in the phase where they like to help, but that comes with a lot of soap and spray. Anything that involves water or any liquid is fun to them. Having homemade cleaners that I know are safe for them to use makes my job in the kitchen easier because I have five little helpers!

The kitchen is an area of our homes that gets a lot of traffic. Whether you're the only chef in your kitchen or have a crowded one like me, making this room safe with natural products is a big step toward a healthier home (and healthier you). In this chapter, you'll find recipes for pretty much every kitchen-related need. Now let's get cookin'!

### Simple Tips to Create a More Sustainable Kitchen

+ Buy in-season produce in bulk and preserve it to save money. My favorite way to preserve produce is by freezing it. It is much easier than canning and doesn't require any special equipment. Simply wash, slice, and store!

✦  Use reusable cloths and tea towels to reduce waste and save money on paper products.

✦  Cook meals from scratch. This may seem like a daunting task, but with a little planning, it will become second nature. At the beginning of the week, I put a variety of frozen meat in a large bowl in my refrigerator to thaw. As soon as the meat is defrosted, I can whip up a healthy meal in no time.

✦  To reduce waste, start a compost pile. Compost is rich in nutrients and can be used in your garden or landscaping soil.

✦  Save all vegetable scraps and peelings in the freezer to throw into your next batch of bone broth. Doing this adds flavor and nutrients and reduces waste.

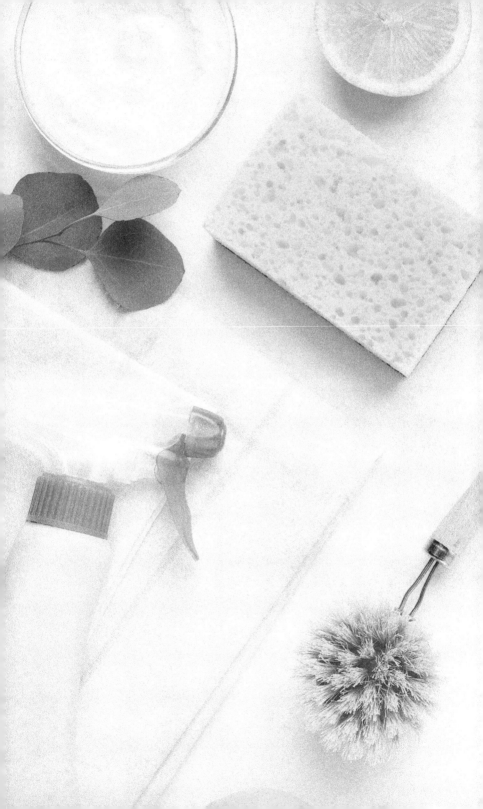

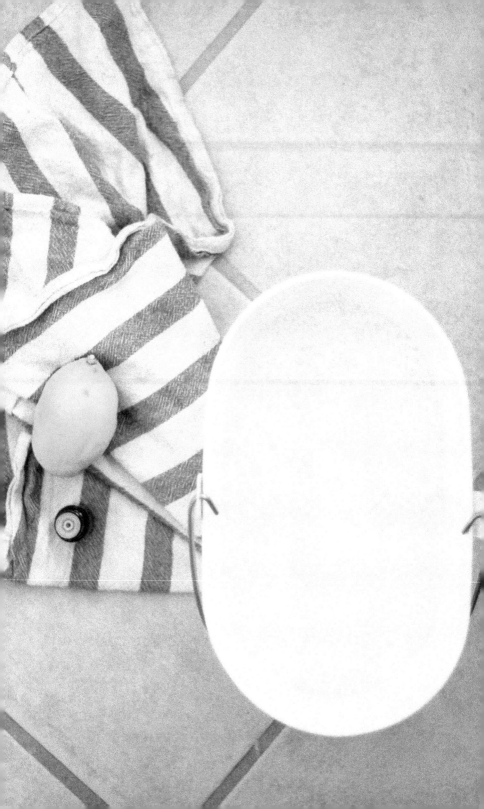

# Lemon Tile Cleaner

Keeping a clean floor is a dream of mine. Keyword: *dream*. With four kids trampling in and out of the house, mopping the floor can seem like a complete waste of time. Even if you don't have kids, if you mop your floor, I'm sure you've noticed how quickly and magically dirt appears. But hey, sometimes it just feels good to restart and stare at a freshly mopped floor, even if it only lasts ten minutes. This all-natural tile cleaner will leave your floors sparkling and smelling lemon-fresh.

## Ingredients

+ ¾ cup baking soda
+ 2 tablespoons salt
+ ¼ cup lemon juice
+ ½ cup vinegar
+ 1 tablespoon castile soap
+ 10 drops lemon essential oil
+ ½ gallon of water
+ A large bucket

## Instructions

1. Combine all the ingredients (except water) into a large bowl or bucket. Stir until well combined.

2. Add about ½ a gallon of water. Swish around to mix.

3. Pour some on the floor and scrub or dip a cloth into the solution and scrub away.

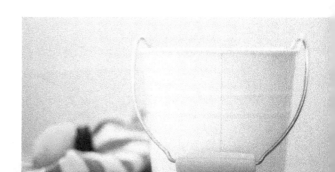

# All-Purpose Spray

Natural cleaning can be easy and inexpensive when you make your products. This DIY all-purpose house cleaner only requires *two* ingredients and works extremely well. Replace all your conventional cleaning products with this simple, natural house cleaner.

This stuff is really all-purpose. Seriously, I use it for almost all of my cleaning. It even works great on mirrors, leaving no streaks.

## Ingredients

+ 16-ounce glass spray bottle
+ 8 ounces vinegar
+ 8 ounces water
+ 20–25 drops lemon essential oil

## Instructions

1. Pour the ingredients into the glass spray bottle.

2. Fill the bottle with water and shake well.

## How to Use

Spray on countertops, bathroom vanities, mirrors, windows, floors, and other surfaces that are soiled. Wipe off with a clean cloth. If you are cleaning something heavily soiled, has soap scum, or hard water stains, allow the mixture to sit for several minutes before wiping clean.

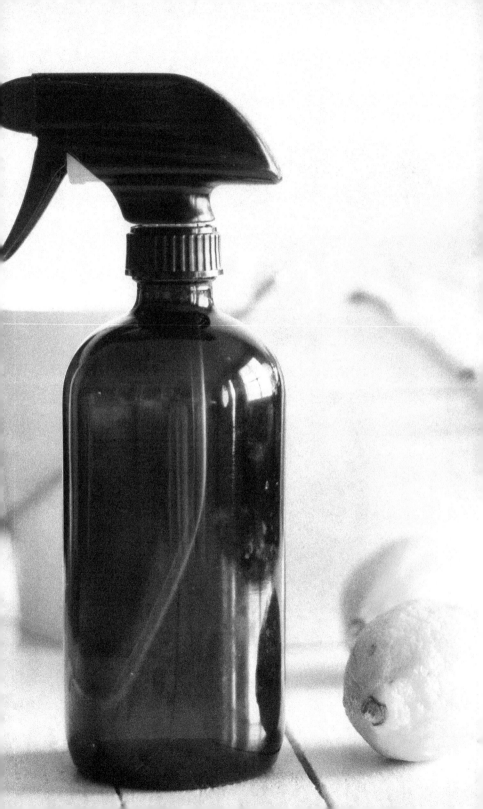

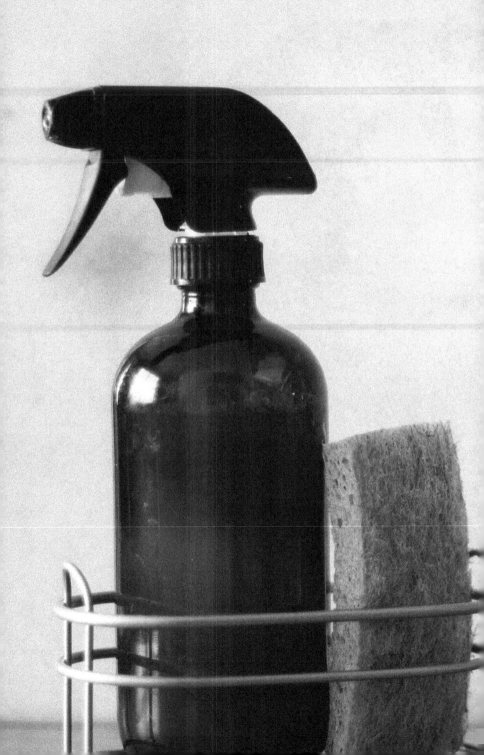

# Granite-Safe Spray

This homemade granite countertop cleaner is so easy to make, safe on natural stone, and works great. This is the best homemade granite cleaner and will help keep your countertops clean and shining. If you have granite in your home, you have to try this three-ingredient all-natural cleaning spray.

When cleaning granite and other natural stone, there are a few ingredients you will want to avoid. Anything with ammonia, vinegar, or bleach could cause damage to granite, marble, and other natural stones if used often.

Overusing harsh chemicals on natural stone can cause it to become dull and break down the sealant.

You will also want to avoid acidic cleaners that contain lemon or lime. However, it is OK to use lemon or lime essential oils because they do not contain citric acid. In fact, lemon is a great option as it is a cleansing essential oil and can add shine.

## Ingredients

+ 1½ cups water
+ ¼ cup rubbing alcohol
+ 1 teaspoon Castile soap
+ 5 drops lemon essential oil
+ 5 drops wild orange essential oil

## Instructions

1. Pour the water, rubbing alcohol, and castile soap into a glass spray bottle.

2. Add in the essential oils.

3. Put the lid on and secure it. Shake well before each use.

# Liquid Dish Soap

I am old fashioned and do my dishes straight in the sink with a little soap and a cloth. I have never seen the point of dishwashers. Maybe I have too many little helpers in the kitchen that like to crawl into the dishwasher while I am emptying or loading it. Whether you use yours or not, having a good all-natural dish soap is a must. I have been using this liquid dish soap for years, and I love the way it works. It cuts grease and leaves the dishes clean and shiny. It's also gentle on your hands and non-toxic. What more can you ask for?

**Ingredients**

+ 16-ounce glass spray bottle
+ ½ cup castile soap
+ 30 drops citrus essential oils

**Instructions**

1. Pour the ingredients into the glass spray bottle.

2. Fill the rest of the bottle with water and shake well.

**Notes**

Citrus essential oils have cleansing and purifying properties, making them great for doing the dishes. You can use one oil or choose a blend of oils. My favorites are grapefruit, lemon, and lime.

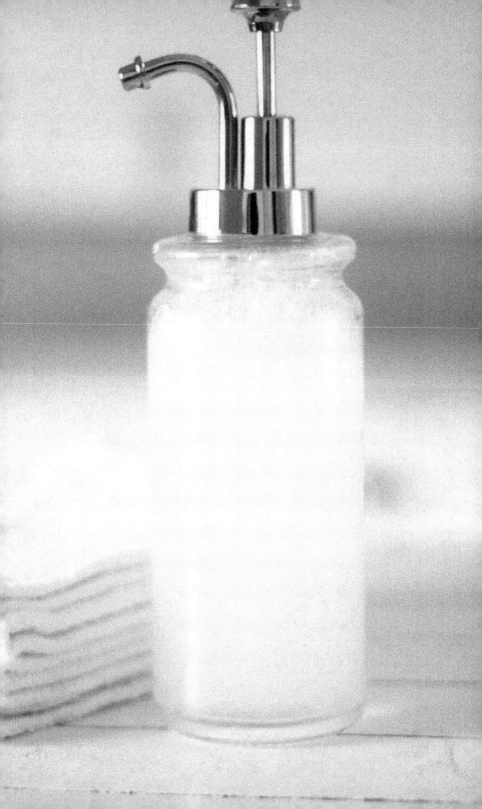

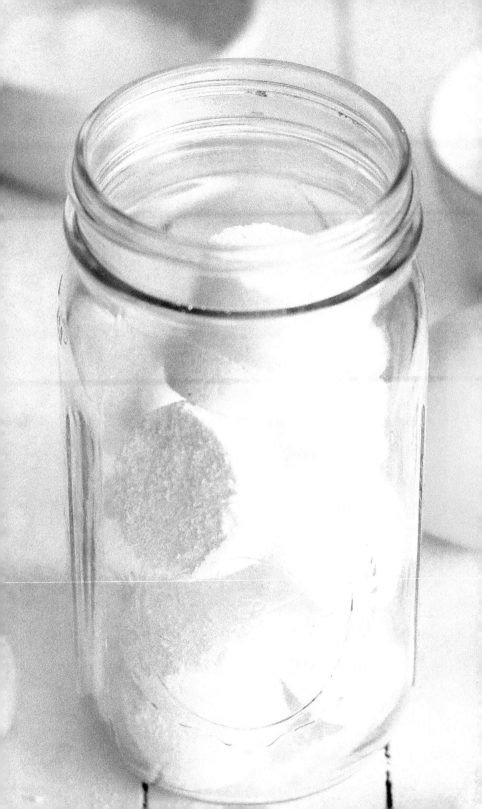

# Dishwasher Tablets

Imagine this. The dishwasher is full of dirty dishes, and you reach under the sink to grab a soap pod . . . and realize you are out. It's barren. Groan. The only thing worse than emptying a clean dishwasher is emptying dirty dishes out of it so that you can hand-wash them. Has this ever happened to you before?

I have found myself in this position one too many times, along with having a full load of dirty clothes and no laundry soap. Times like these leave me digging around to see what I can find in my house to make do. These little emergencies have brought me many new DIY recipes that I still use today. And now, reader, I gift them to you as well. You're welcome.

The best part? These homemade products are always all-natural and usually work just as well as the "real thing." These DIY dishwasher soap pods are simple to make and work incredibly well. They are made with all-natural ingredients to help keep toxins out of your home.

## Ingredients

+ 1 cup washing soda
+ 1 cup borax
+ ¼ cup Epsom salt
+ ¼ cup vinegar (you can also use lemon juice)
+ 20–25 drops lemon essential oil

## Instructions

1. Mix all your dry ingredients in a medium-size mixing bowl.

2. Pour the vinegar over the dry ingredients. Once the bubbles go down, stir well.

3. Add lemon essential oil and stir well.

4. Transfer the mixture to an ice cube tray or silicone molds. Press the mixture down into the molds.

5.   Allow the molds to sit overnight to make sure it is completely dry
     and then pop the mixture out of the molds. (If you are in a hurry
     and need it right away, you can put 1 tablespoon of this powder
     into the dishwasher without it being dry, and it will still work
     just fine.)

# Stainless Steel Spray

It can be hard to keep any stainless steel appliance clean and smudge-free. Little fingers love to touch as many surfaces as possible. This is another reason why it is important to use natural cleaners in your home with little ones. Remember that nothing is off-limits and will most likely end up in their mouth at some point. This stainless steel spray takes less than two minutes to whip up and helps keep your appliances smudge-free.

## Ingredients

+ Spray bottle
+ Water
+ Vinegar
+ Lemon essential oil
+ Orange essential oil

## Instructions

1. Mix equal parts water and vinegar into a glass spray bottle.

2. Add in essential oils.

3. Shake well before each use.

4. Spray straight on the surface and wipe clean with a microfiber cloth.

### Notes

If using a 16-ounce spray bottle, you can use 12–15 drops of essential oils. Adjust the amount according to the size bottle you are using.

# Stainless Steel Polish

This polish can be used after the stainless steel spray or for touchups. This comes in handy when you find fingerprints or a smudge on the appliance, and you want a quick shine.

**Ingredients**

+ ⅛ cup olive oil
+ 5 drops tea tree essential oil

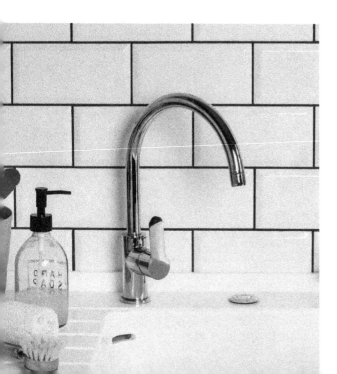

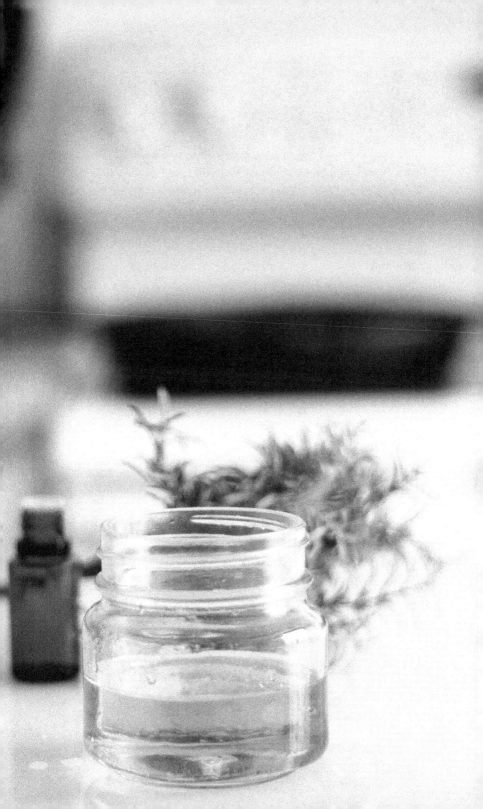

# Oven Cleaner

The last thing I want to put in my oven is harsh cleaners filled with chemicals. They give me an instant headache, and they seem to linger when I am cooking days later. I started experimenting with my favorite natural cleaners and finally came up with a solution that works. This took a bit of testing, and I almost resorted back to conventional cleaners out of frustration. Every time I tried to come up with an oven cleaner, it involved so much elbow grease I could barely get the job done. This three-step process makes it so much easier to remove tough stains.

You may expect something elaborate after all the time I spent experimenting, but this is not. All you need is vinegar, baking soda, water, and salt. It's the three-step process that is key in this recipe.

## Ingredients

+ ½ cup baking soda
+ 3 tablespoons water
+ Soft brush or cleaning cloth
+ Salt
+ 2 cups vinegar
+ 1 cup water
+ 10 drops lemon essential oil (optional)

## Instructions

### Step 1

1. Remove baking racks from the oven. Those are best to wash separately.

2. Mix the baking soda and water until it forms a paste.

3. Apply the paste all over the oven, avoiding the heating elements, using a soft scrub brush or a cleaning cloth.

4. Let the mixture sit for 4 hours or until dry.

## Step 2

1. Sprinkle salt over the baking soda.

2. Remove the baking soda with a dry cleaning cloth. The salt will help to loosen grime and stains.

## Step 3

1. Combine vinegar, water, and essential oils into a spray bottle.

2. Spray the liquid mixture all over the oven.

3. Wipe away the remaining baking soda and salt with a cloth.

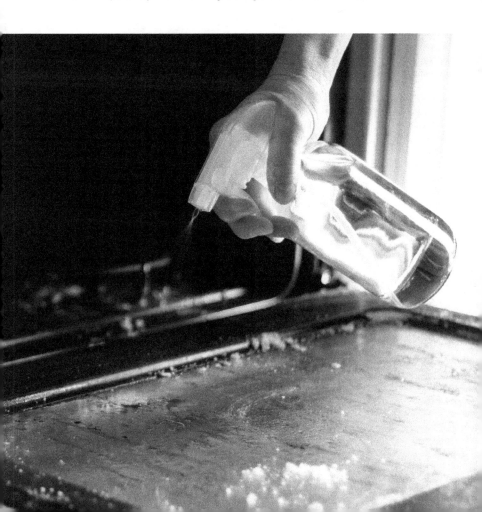

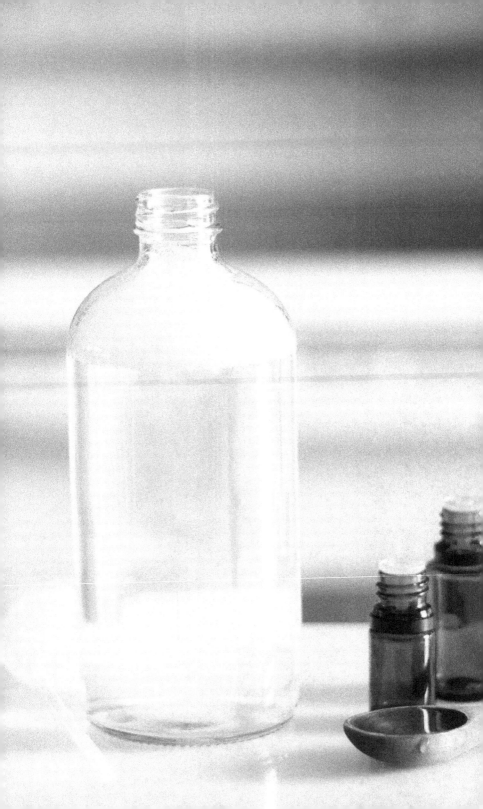

# Degreaser Spray

If you've cooked anything ever, you'll know that sometimes a little degreaser spray is necessary for the kitchen. This spray can come in handy when doing the dishes, cleaning, or even hand washing. I have even used this spray as a spot treatment when I had an oil splash on my clothes. (So if you're looking for a multipurpose recipe to try, this one is your friend.)

I use Sals Sud in this recipe and, though it is similar to castile soap, the key difference is that Sals Sud is a powerful natural cleaner and gentle on the skin. Now let's get de-greasing.

**Ingredients**

+ 1 teaspoon Sals Sud
+ ¼ cup vinegar
+ 1 cup water
+ 10 drops lemon essential oil
+ 10 drops wild orange essential oil

**Instructions**

1. Add all the ingredients to a glass spray bottle.

2. Shake well before each use.

3. Spray on the area of concern and let it sit for a few minutes. Wipe the surface clean with warm water.

# Fruit and Veggie Wash

Before I had kids, washing my produce wasn't something I usually did. I didn't think it mattered. Well, then I did a little research and realized just how important this was.

Just like everything in this book, I especially love that this spray is made with all-natural ingredients, so I don't have to worry about adding more chemicals to my food. I buy a lot of my produce organic, but not everything.

If organic foods aren't in the budget, then you should consider using this spray. Though washing your produce isn't going to get all the pesticides off, it will most certainly help.

**Ingredients**

+ Filtered water
+ 1 cup white vinegar
+ 10 drops lemon essential oil

**Instructions**

1. Add the vinegar and lemon essential oil to a 16-ounce glass spray bottle.

2. Top off with water and shake well before use.

3. Spray each piece of produce and scrub gently with a scrub brush or your hands.

4. Rinse with water.

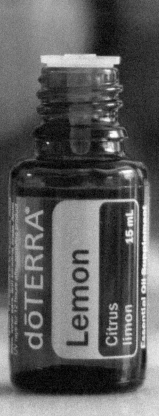

# Beeswax Covers

I try my best to reduce plastic and foil use in my home. I don't like the extra waste, and I don't want those things touching my food. I have silicone lids that fit on any size bowl that I love, but before this recipe, I only had two.

Instead of going out and buying more, I decided to make my own. I found that making beeswax covers are simple, cost-effective, and produce zero waste. All you need for this project is beeswax and some fabric. It is best to use an organic fabric, but any fabric will do.

You will also need a paintbrush or a piece of cardboard to spread the beeswax onto the cloth. Fair warning: beeswax isn't easy to get off of things, so I suggest using something you don't mind throwing away or designating specifically to your beeswax projects.

## Materials

+ Fabric, cut into squares or circles
+ Beeswax pellets or a block
+ Scissors
+ Paintbrush or cardboard

## Instructions

1. Preheat the oven to 175 degrees.

2. Cut fabric into squares or circles. You can use the plates, bowls, or baking pans you already own as your templates.

3. Place the fabric pieces on a baking dish covered with parchment paper.

4. Sprinkle beeswax over the fabric. If you are using a block of beeswax, you will need to shred it over the fabric.

5.  Bake for about 5 minutes or until the beeswax is melted.
    Spread the beeswax evenly on the fabric with the paintbrush or
    cardboard piece.

6.  Allow it to dry completely.

## How to Use

When you place the fabric over a bowl, plate, or dish, *press down*. The
heat from your hands will slightly melt the wax to seal to the bowl and
keep food covered.

**Notes**

To clean the fabric, hand wash it in cold water. If you use warm water,
it can melt the wax. Hang to dry and reuse. After a while, you may
need to add another coat of beeswax if you notice they aren't clinging
as well as they used to.

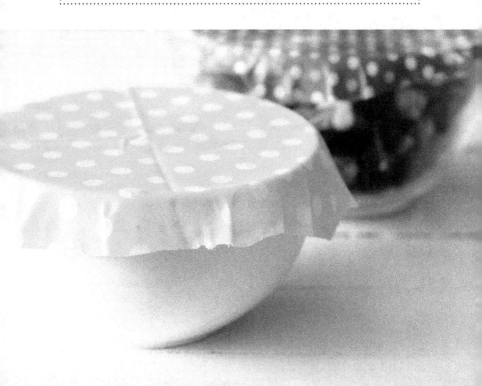

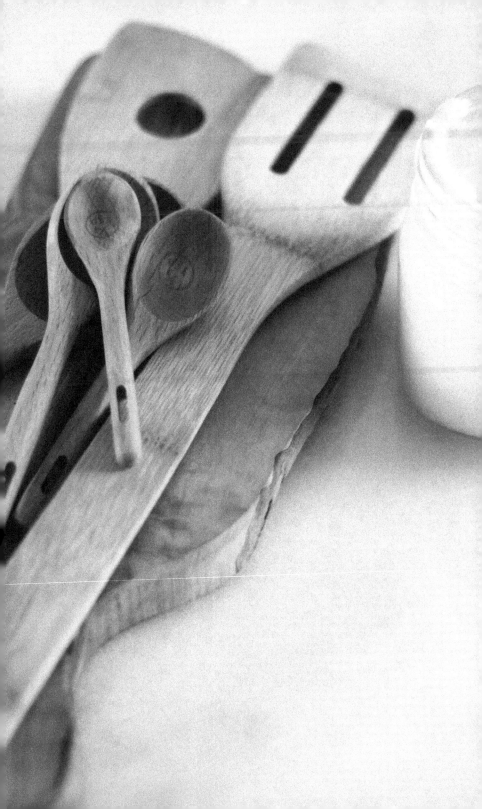

# Homemade Wooden Spoon Butter

We use a lot of wooden utensils in my home for cooking. It is either wood, stainless steel, or cast iron over here. I got rid of all the plastic and Teflon years ago. (I hate the idea of warming and storing food in plastic due to the toxic chemicals found in them.) I love a cast-iron skillet and a wooden spoon because they get better with time. Wooden utensils don't need much care, but to prevent them from cracking or splitting, you may want to rub them down with some spoon butter now and then. It is also important to dry wooden utensils, rolling pins, and wood cutting boards completely after washing them.

Spoon butter can be made with any oil and beeswax. I am using coconut oil in this recipe, but you could also use olive oil, avocado oil, almond oil, or sunflower oil. After several washes, I will massage a little spoon of butter into the utensils, and then they are as good as new. You won't need a lot when you use spoon butter on your wooden utensils, and you can wipe the butter off with a clean cloth before using it the next time if you wish.

## Ingredients

+ 2 tablespoons beeswax pellets
+ 8 tablespoons coconut oil

## Instructions

1. Melt the ingredients in a double boiler.

2. Allow it to cool slightly and then transfer to a mason jar or another airtight container for storage.

### Notes

The mixture will harden as it cools and have a "buttery" consistency.

## Kitchen Diffuser Blends

Picture this: a clean kitchen, windows open with a warm breeze blowing through, dinner prepped, and the diffuser pumping out a fresh, clean lemon smell. Okay, I admit, this is not the reality most days, but a girl can dream, can't she? I seriously can't think of anything better than a clean kitchen with a diffuser going. Having a diffuser in the kitchen is the best, trust me on this one.

I love diffusing essential oils all over my home, but the kitchen is my favorite place, probably because it is where I spend the most time. I like to keep the smell simple, fresh, and clean. I usually pick a citrus oil or two to keep moods uplifted. In a house full of kids, this is a must.

Here are some of my favorite blends for the kitchen:

### Clean Kitchen

4 drops lemon
4 drops rosemary

### Bright Kitchen

3 drops lemon
3 drops wild orange
2 drops sweet fennel

### Fresh Kitchen

3 drops lime
3 drops cypress
2 drops wild orange

### Apple Pie

3 drops cinnamon
2 drops clove
2 drops cardamom

### Sugar Cookie

3 drops cinnamon
2 drops wild orange
2 drops clove

### Citrus Bliss

3 drops grapefruit
2 drops lemon
2 drops wild orange

### Minty Fresh

4 drops lemon
4 drops peppermint

### Spotless Kitchen

3 drops wild orange
2 drops lime
2 drops eucalyptus

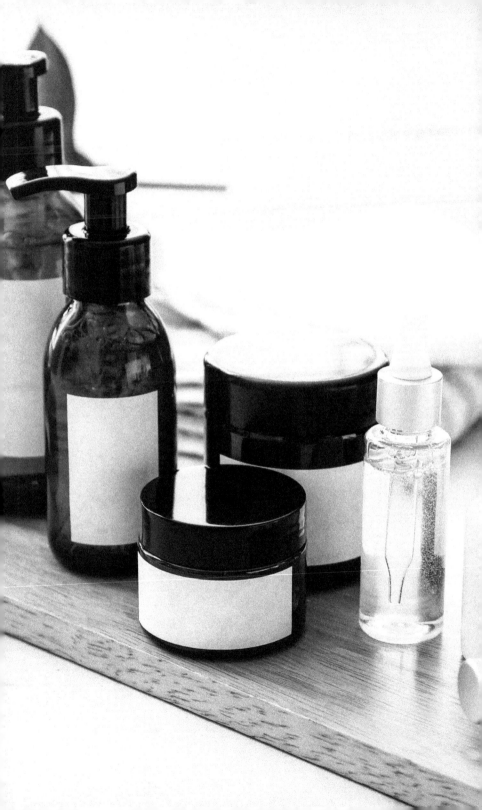

# CHAPTER 2

# Natural Bathroom Remedies

Believe it or not, the bathroom is getting its own chapter in this book. Obviously, we will be talking about natural cleaners, but other common bathroom products will be covered too. I will even share some diffuser blends that can help to purify and cover odor. This chapter will show you how you can replace conventional cleaners with all-natural ones that actually work. I am a huge neat-freak; however, even though my standards have lowered with the more kids I have, having a clean bathroom is still on the top of my list.

Every time the kids come out of the bathroom, I find towels on the floor, rugs disheveled, and water spots on the mirrors. Oh, how I love them dearly, but seriously, how do the messes happen so fast? I love that I can leave my cleaners out and unlocked for quick little wipe downs that need to happen multiple times a day.

**Simple Tips to Create a More Sustainable Bathroom**

+ Make the switch to reusable soap dispensers to cut down on waste and to save money!

+ Make your haircare and skincare products. You will find some of my favorite recipes in later chapters. Not only will this save money and reduce waste, but it is also much healthier for you.

+ Use natural cleaning products stored in plastic-free refillable containers.

# Glass Cleaner

I'm one of those strange birds who actually loves to clean. One thing I can't stand is streaks on a mirror or window. Before I was a "crunchy mom," I used a lot of Windex. So that's why glass cleaner was one of the first things I knew I had to switch out when I was going to all-natural, but I wasn't happy about it. I was worried I wouldn't be able to come up with something that would leave my glass streak-free and sparkling like the store-bought kind. You have likely had some of the same misgivings as well.

Thankfully, we are both wrong! Early on in my journey, I found out that making my own glass cleaner was easy, and I was amazed at how well it worked. I love that it is all-natural, so I don't have to worry about breathing in the fumes or my kids finding and playing with it. In fact, the kids can now help me clean the mirrors in the bathroom after they splatter them with toothpaste and water multiple times a day.

All you need for this cleaner is vinegar, rubbing alcohol, water, and essential oils.

## Ingredients

+ 1 cup vinegar
+ 1 cup distilled water
+ ⅛ cup rubbing alcohol
+ 10 drops lemon essential oil
+ 10 drops lavender essential oil

## Instructions

1. Add all the ingredients to a glass spray bottle.

2. Shake before each use.

3. Spray onto glass and wipe off with a paper towel or microfiber cloth.

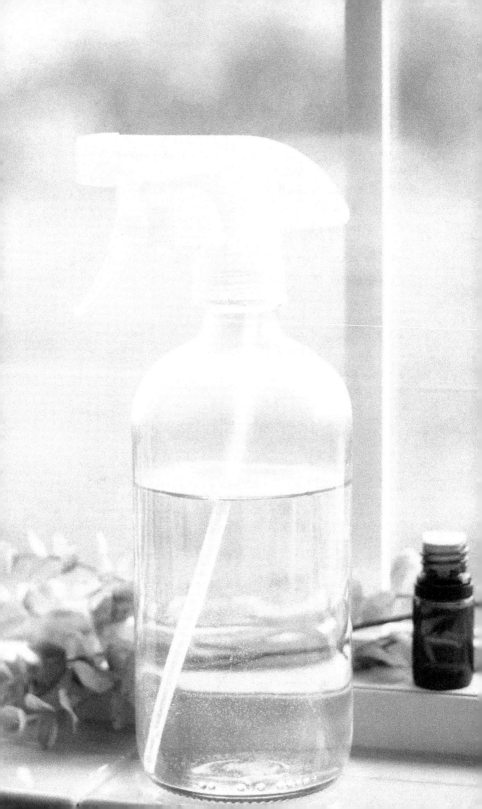

# Bathroom Floor Scrub

Vinegar and baking soda are great cleaners for tile and grout. Did I mention that I use a whole lot of baking soda and vinegar when cleaning? If you don't love the smell of vinegar, I suggest you diffuse some lemon essential oil on cleaning day. It will overpower the vinegar smell and leave your house smelling fresh and clean.

If you have natural stone tile, you can replace the vinegar with rubbing alcohol, as vinegar can damage natural stone over time.

## Ingredients

+ Baking soda
+ Water
+ Vinegar (or rubbing alcohol)
+ Tea tree essential oil

**Notes**

I am not giving exact amounts in the ingredient list because it depends on your bathroom size. Besides, this recipe doesn't have to be exact, anyway; this is one you can totally wing and it will still turn out great. Continue to the directions for more guidance.

## Instructions

1. The first step to cleaning any floor is sweeping it. There's nothing worse (or more ineffective) than mopping around dirt and crumbs.

2. Mix the baking soda and water in a bowl until a thick paste is formed. It should be about ⅓ cup water to 1 cup baking soda.

3. Slather the baking soda paste into the grout. Allow it to sit for a couple of minutes or until it is dry.

4.  Mix equal parts of vinegar and water in a spray bottle. Add in the tea tree essential oil—I use about 15 drops for a 16-ounce glass spray bottle.

5.  Spray the vinegar mixture onto the floor and wipe clean with a mop or cloth.

6.  You may need to spend a lot of extra time on the grout to get the baking soda to come up. After all the baking soda is up, you may want to spray again with the vinegar mixture to add extra shine.

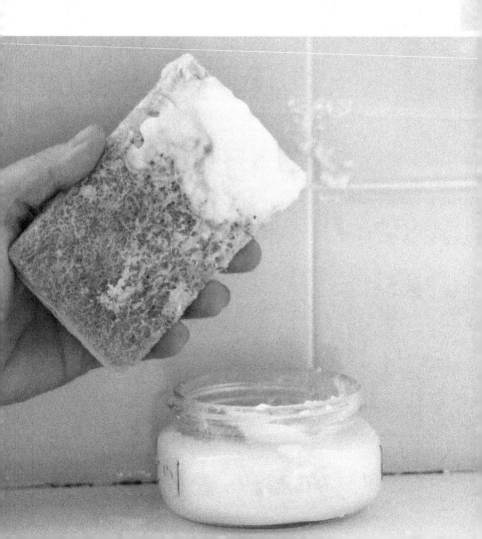

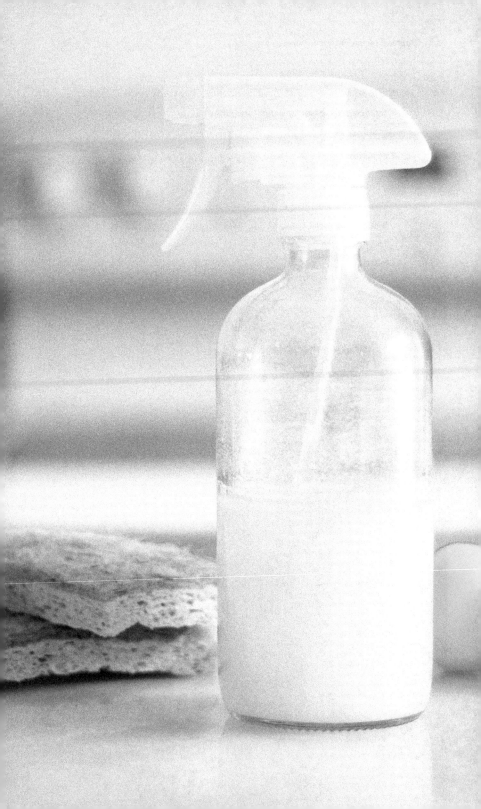

# Mold and Mildew Cleaner

Mold and mildew are pretty much going to happen in your bathroom at some point. However, what you might not know if those store-bought cleaners designed to remove them can be just as harmful as the mold and mildew itself. Luckily, making your own spray to remove these inevitable visitors is easy and effective. It is made with safe ingredients, but it is still best to wear a mask when removing mold. This will prevent you from breathing in any in the process.

## Ingredients

+ 1 cup vinegar
+ 30 drops tea tree essential oil
+ 15 drops lemon essential oil
+ Glass spray bottle

## Instructions

1. Mix all the ingredients in a glass spray bottle.

2. Shake well before each use.

## How to Use

1. Spray the mixture on the area of concern.

2. Allow it to sit for 15 minutes.

3. Wipe clean with a cloth.

# Easy Homemade Toothpaste

Have you ever read the warning label on the back of your toothpaste tube? Mine says, "Keep out of reach of children. If more is swallowed than the normal amount used for brushing, get medical help or contact poison control right away."

*Yikes!* Something that my kids see me put in my mouth could greatly harm them if they put it in their mouth. This is why I decided to make my own toothpaste with natural and safe ingredients.

**Ingredients**

- ✦ Calcium carbonate
- ✦ Xylitol
- ✦ Baking soda
- ✦ Coconut oil
- ✦ Essential oils

**Instructions**

1. Mix 5 parts calcium carbonate, 3 parts xylitol, and 2 parts baking soda in a bowl.

2. Add 5 drops clove bud and 15 drops peppermint essential oil. (Or check out other essential oils you can use below.)

3. Add 4 parts coconut oil and mix until well combined.

4. Store your toothpaste in an airtight container. Simple.

**Notes**

You can make any quantity you want. I do this with tablespoon amounts and usually double this recipe.

## Best Essential Oils for Homemade Toothpaste

1. **Peppermint**: Add peppermint essential oil to help freshen breath and leave the mouth feeling clean.

2. **Spearmint**: Spearmint doesn't have as strong a mint flavor as peppermint, and my kids prefer it. I add a few drops of this into their toothpaste to freshen breath.

3. **Clove**: Everyone should add a few drops of clove to their homemade toothpaste. Clove has powerful cleansing and purifying properties.

4. **Wild Orange**: Wild orange will help cleanse the mouth.

5. **Cinnamon**: Cinnamon essential oil can be used to freshen breath and naturally whiten teeth.

# Homemade Mouthwash

I like fresh breath as much as the next, but when I read the label on my store-bought mouthwash, it went straight into the trash. Mouthwash is high in sodium and may be doing more harm than good for your overall health.

Your mouth is full of beneficial bacteria that your body needs. In fact, it is the body's first defense against illness. By overusing conventional mouthwash, you can kill the good bacteria in your mouth that you need for overall wellness.

This homemade spearmint mouthwash will leave your breath fresh and will help to cleanse and purify your mouth. Homemade mouthwash is simple to make, and once you start using it, you will never want to go back to conventional.

Some of my favorite essential oils to keep my breath fresh and my mouth cleansed are spearmint, peppermint, wintergreen, and wild orange.

### Ingredients

+ 1 cup of filtered water
+ 1 teaspoon baking soda
+ 5 drops of pure essential oil
+ 10 drops of mineral drops, optional

### Instructions

1. Pour the water into an airtight glass container.

2. Add in baking soda, essential oils, and mineral drops if using.

3. Secure lid and shake well.

4. Swish about 2 tablespoons around in your mouth for 15 seconds and then spit out.

# DIY Hand Sanitizer Spray

This spray is something I have been making and using for seven years. It is probably one of my most used DIYs. This homemade hand sanitizer spray should be in everyone's purse, diaper bag, house, and car. Thankfully, it is cost-effective and takes less than two minutes to whip up.

Conventional sanitizing sprays typically contain chemicals that can be harmful if swallowed and can dry out the skin if overused. When we use conventional hand sanitizing spray, we kill off the bacteria that we need to build a healthy immune system. Overusing products with antibacterial agents can make our bodies immune to them, and then when we need them when we are actually sick, they may not be as effective.

Switching to a natural spray won't do this. Your body can't build up a resistance to essential oils, so this hand sanitizer spray is a great option for keeping germs away.

**Ingredients**

+ 2 tablespoon rubbing alcohol or witch hazel
+ 3 drops each of cinnamon, clove, eucalyptus, rosemary, and wild orange essential oil
+ 1 tsp fractionated coconut oil (optional)
+ 2-ounce glass spray bottle

**Instructions**

1. Add all the ingredients to the spray bottle.

2. Top off with water.

3. Shake well before each use.

4. Spray on hands and rub together. Or spray on a surface and wipe.

# Reusable Cleaning Wipes

I love having these cleaning wipes available for my family to use. Having safe, natural options allows all my kids to help on cleaning day, and I don't have to worry about them being exposed to harmful chemicals.

These wipes are great for wiping down tables and chairs after mealtime, taking off makeup, and wiping down the countertops, bathroom vanities, or toys. You can use them to clean toys because if you have kids anything like mine, they put *everything* in their mouths. I like knowing these are made with non-toxic ingredients, and it is okay if my youngest ones get this in their mouths. Even if you don't have kids, think about wiping down frequently touched items like your phone or quickly wipe surfaces like doorknobs and faucet handles.

## Ingredients

+ 2 cups warm water
+ 2 tablespoons fractionated coconut oil
+ 3 drops wild orange essential oil
+ 2 drops lemon essential oil
+ 2 drops clove essential oil
+ 1 tablespoon of Castile soap
+ Clean cloths

## Instructions

### Option 1

1. Add the ingredients into a glass spray bottle.

2. Spray this on a surface or even directly onto dirty hands and wipe off with a clean washcloth.

3. You can also spray it straight on the clean washcloth and then wipe the surface (or hands) with the cloth.

## Option 2

1.   Add all the ingredients to an airtight container, such as a Tupperware bowl or mason jar.

2.   Place about 5–8 reusable wipes in the container. Push them below to the liquid to make sure they are wet.

3.   Seal the container.

After a few days, you can wash the reusable cloths and make a new mixture.

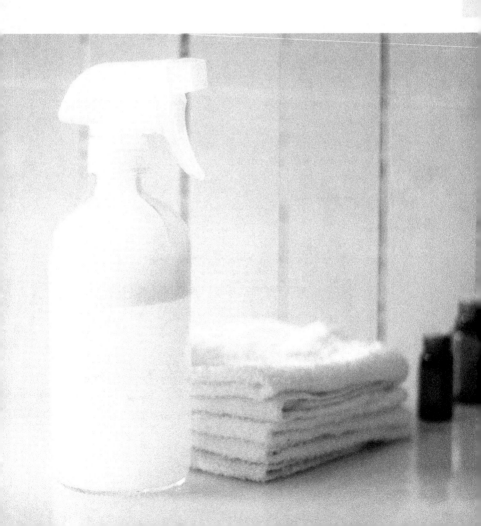

# Tub and Sink Soft Scrub

I often stick to my all-purpose spray for everyday cleaning, but sometimes I have to break out the soft scrub for more stubborn stains. This stuff is the non-toxic version of the Comet cleaner.

You can use this scrub for a deeper clean or when dealing with rust, rings, stains, and hard water. We tend to have hard water in our home, and this stuff works like magic to remove it. With this homemade shower cleaner recipe, it's now easy to have a sparkling bathroom.

I find lemon essential oil to work the best in this recipe, but if you don't have it, you can replace it with wild orange, tea tree, lavender, or rosemary. All of these essential oils are great for cleaning.

## Ingredients

+ 1 cup baking soda
+ ¼ cup castile soap
+ 2 tablespoon Hydrogen Peroxide
+ 10 drops lemon essential oil
+ Airtight container

## Instructions

1. Pour the baking soda into the airtight container.

2. Add in castile soap, hydrogen peroxide, and essential oil.

3. Stir well and close the lid.

## How to Use It

1. The mixture will be pretty thick, so you will have to scoop it out with your hands. Spread a generous amount all over the tub, paying extra attention to grout and stubborn stains.

2. Let it sit for a few minutes to soak in.

3. Wipe off with a cloth. For tough stains, you may want to use a scrub brush and scrub it vigorously for several minutes before wiping with a cloth.

4. Turn the shower (or sink) on to rinse it out.

**Notes**

I find it best to make a new batch before each cleaning, as it doesn't hold up well long-term. This amount will clean the three tubs in my home.

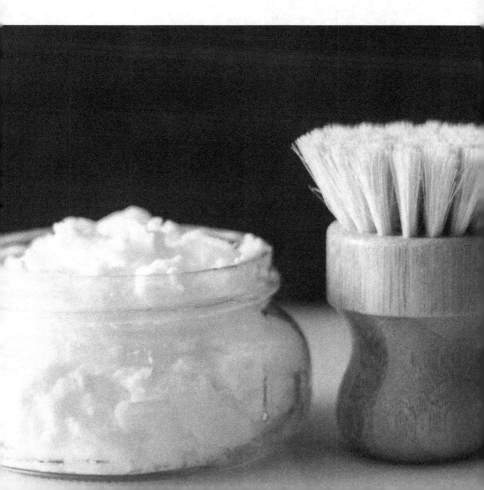

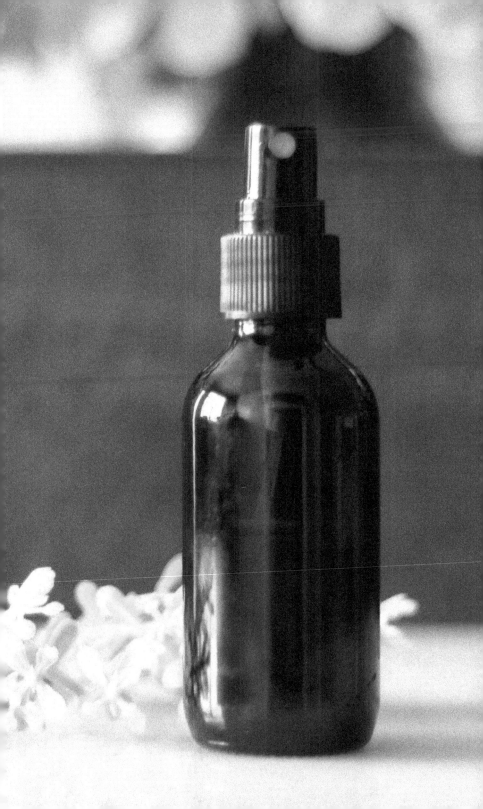

# Poo-Pourri Spray

This is something all bathrooms need—am I right? After you clean the bathroom, it doesn't take much time until it is smelly again! This spray can help keep yours smelling fresh and clean longer. I love using my essential oils to make air fresheners like this. You will see more recipes with them throughout the book because they work great and are all-natural. I hate spraying toxins into the air to "freshen" it. That doesn't make much sense to me.

This spray is easy to make (the golden rule) and only requires a few ingredients. You can spray it straight into the air or into the toilet bowl. It can be used as needed.

## Ingredients

- 4-ounce glass spray bottle
- 30 drops essential oil (my favorite blends are in the next section)
- 2 teaspoons of vegetable glycerin
- 2 tablespoons witch hazel
- Distilled water, as needed

## Instructions

1. Add the essential oils, vegetable glycerin, and witch hazel to the spray bottle.

2. Shake well to combine ingredients.

3. Fill the rest of the bottle with water.

## Essential Oil Blends to Try for a Natural Bathroom

### Fresh

10 drops lemon
10 drops rosemary
10 drops spearmint

### Citrus

10 drops lemon
10 drops lime
10 drops wild orange

### Floral

10 drops lavender
10 drops jasmine
10 drops patchouli

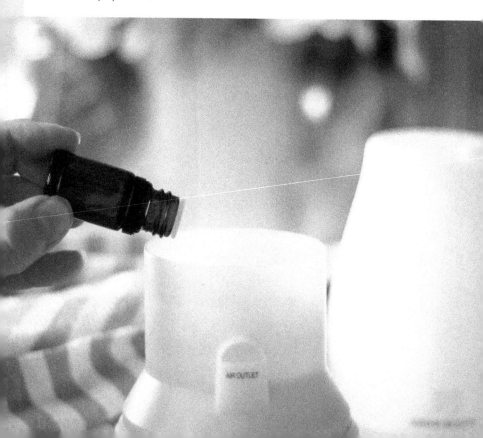

## Bathroom Diffuser Blends

You know you are truly "the crazy oil lady" when you have a diffuser in the bathroom. But for real, a diffuser in the bathroom is a great idea and one of the places in your home that needs it the most. I love diffusing essential oils in my home to help with mood, support immune systems, and cover up odor. I have a house full of boys, so the last one is a must.

These bathroom diffuser blends will leave the bathroom smelling fresh and clean, even when it is not, and can make a calming atmosphere for a luxurious spa night at home.

### Clean Bathroom

3 drops lemon
3 drops tea tree
2 drops spearmint

### Fresh Bathroom

5 drops eucalyptus
4 drops peppermint
2 drops rosemary

### Spa Day

4 drops bergamot
3 drops sandalwood
2 drops ylang-ylang

### Odor Buster

5 drops lemon
4 drops lime
3 drops Siberian fir

### Bath Time

5 drops lavender
3 drops chamomile
2 drops wild orange
2 drops rose

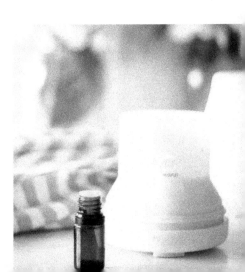

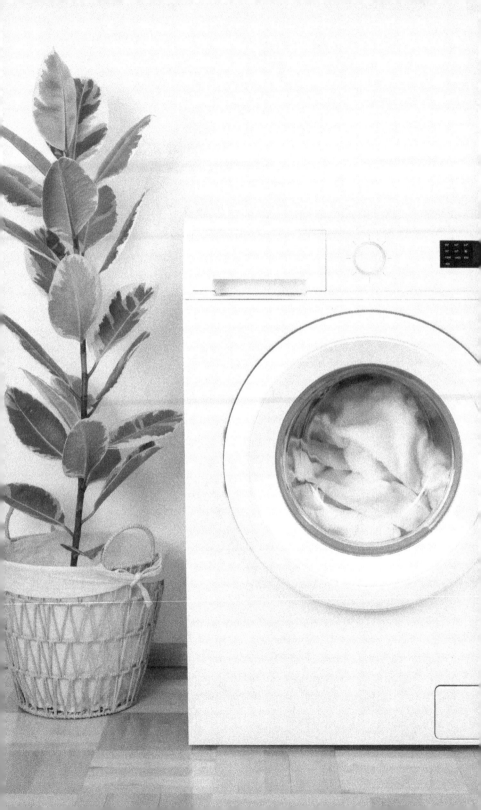

# CHAPTER 3

# Natural Laundry Remedies

I have been making my own laundry products since I got married, and it has saved us so much money over the past eight years. Sometimes I like to walk through the laundry aisle at the grocery store just to see how much money I am saving—it is satisfying. Soon, you'll be able to have the same experience.

To give you an idea of how much more economical it is, you can make five gallons of laundry soap for less than two dollars and can whip up your own dryer sheets with just vinegar and old t-shirts. On the other hand, a large Tide container only brings four pounds of product and is almost twenty dollars. Considering how often we all need to do laundry, you will soon see the financial benefits of choosing natural laundry products. Believe me when I say these recipes are tried and true.

It is normal for my kids to come in for the day covered in mud, grass stains, and leftover dinner. My boys are obsessed with working in the garage with their daddy, so a little grease and grime can be added to the list. If you like to garden, have sweaty workout sessions, or simply need safe and effective laundry products for everyday use, you will find all-natural alternatives in this chapter for all of your laundry needs to help eliminate toxins from your clothes, towels, and home.

### Simple Laundry Tips

+ Do a load a day so you don't get behind. With a large family, the laundry can pile up quickly and become overwhelming. Keeping up with it makes it much more manageable.

+ Let the kids help. My little ones fold and put away all of their own clothes. No, it isn't perfect, but it teaches responsibility and gives me one less job to do. As long as the clothes make it into the right dresser, I am happy.

+ We don't get fancy with sorting over here. Unless it is something really nice, it all gets washed together. We skip the laundry baskets and hampers and throw dirty clothes straight into the washer. At the end of the day, I run a load, and it is ready to fold by morning.

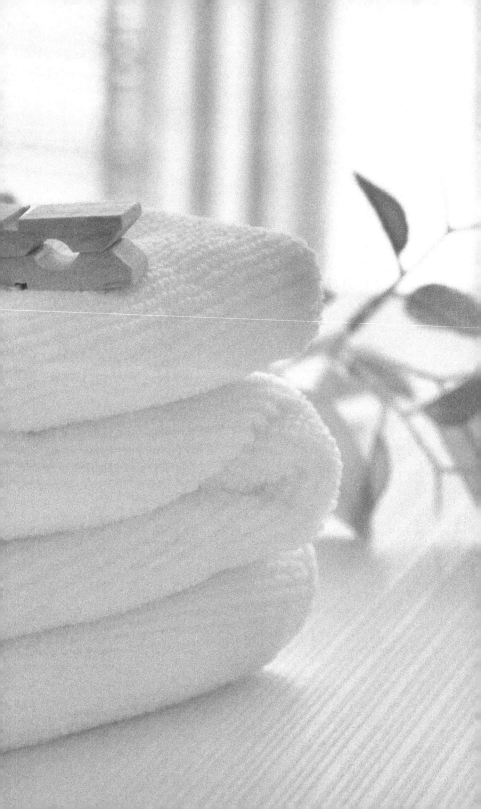

# Liquid Laundry Soap

Making laundry soap is a great place to start trying to get rid of conventional items from your home. It's easy, works instantly, and is extremely cost-effective. If you still have some detergent leftover in your home as you read this, that's OK. Just use it up and save the container; you can store this new all-natural version inside it once it's empty!

It takes less than twenty minutes from start to finish to make five gallons of all-natural laundry soap. You can even use your choice of essential oils to fit the scent you are looking for.

## Ingredients

+ 1 cup borax
+ ½ cup washing soda (can be found in the laundry section)
+ 1 Fels Naptha soap bar, 5 ounces
+ 5-gallon bucket with lid
+ Cheese grater (I keep one in the laundry room and have a different one for the kitchen)
+ 30–50 drops of essential oils of choice

## Instructions

1. Add ½ gallon of water to your bucket. Stir in borax and washing soda.

2. Shred your soap bar with the cheese grater—melt soap shreds in 1 cup of water over medium heat. Stir often.

3. Add melted soap to the bucket and stir well.

4. Add essential oil(s) of choice.

5. Fill the bucket the rest of the way with room-temperature tap water. Stir until all ingredients are well combined.

6. Let sit overnight and then shake bucket well the next day.

**Notes**

I like to pour the detergent in a ½ gallon jar for easier handling. You can also store it in your old laundry soap containers. Shake well before each use. Use ½ cup of detergent per load. This soap will keep for up to six months.

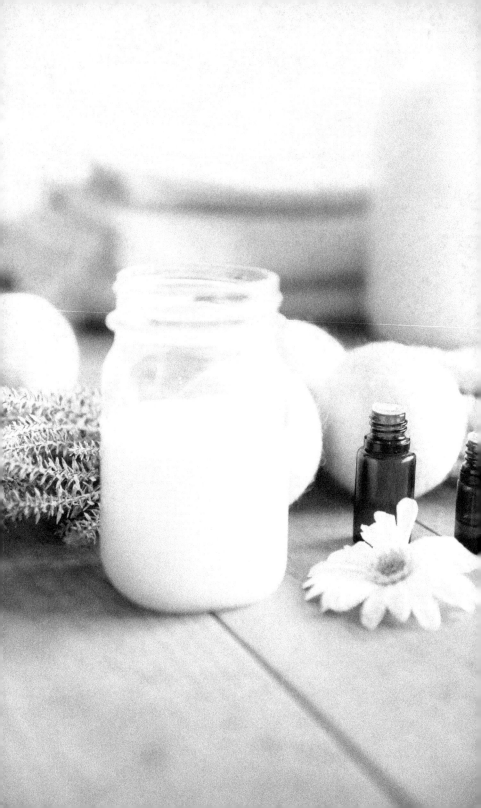

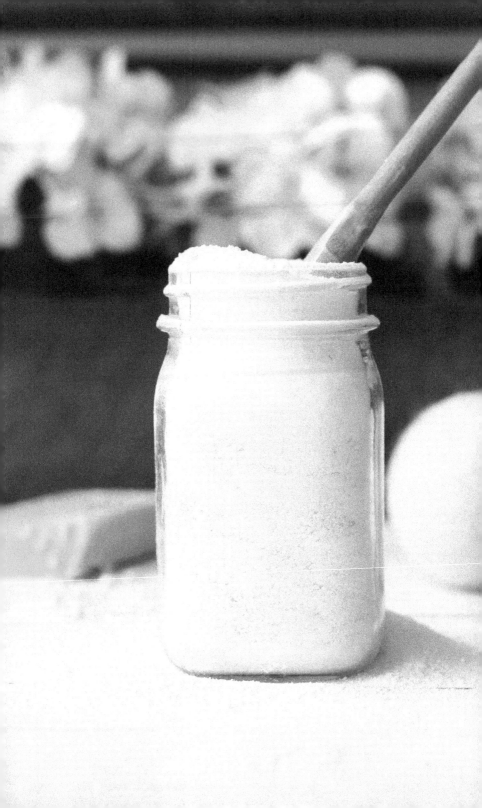

# Powder Laundry Soap

When I first started my blog, my homemade laundry soap was one of the first things I shared. I have been using that exact recipe for over seven years, and I love that I can make five gallons for less than two dollars. Talk about a money saver! After multiple requests from my readers, I now have a homemade powder laundry soap recipe for those who prefer this form over liquid.

This recipe uses similar ingredients to the liquid soap, making it cost-effective, too.

It is sensitive enough to be used with baby clothes, delicates, and even cloth diapers! You only need a couple of tablespoons per load.

## Ingredients

+ 1 bar castile soap (or Fels Naptha soap bar)
+ 2 cups washing soda
+ 2 cups baking soda
+ 30 drops lavender essential oil (optional)

## Instructions

1. Finely grate the soap bar using a cheese grater.

2. Add the shredded soap bar, washing soda, and baking soda to a large mixing bowl.

3. Stir until well combined

4. Add in essential oils.

5. Store in an airtight container.

**Notes**

Use 2 tablespoons per load. This soap is safe to use in high-efficiency washers. I store mine in a half-gallon glass mason jar, and I keep a tablespoon measuring spoon in the container to make it easy to measure. This recipe will keep for one year.

## Best Essential Oils for Laundry Soap

1.  **Lavender:** Lavender is a calming, relaxing essential oil with a lovely floral smell. This one is my favorite for laundry soap.

2.  **Wild Orange:** Invigorating, uplifting, and cleansing; wild orange is perfect for your laundry soap. It adds a fresh scent to your clean clothes.

3.  **Melaleuca:** Melaleuca is a purifying and cleansing essential oil. If you've ever forgotten to put wet laundry straight in the dryer when it is done, add 2–3 drops to the wet clothes before putting them in the dryer.

4.  **Peppermint:** If you like a fresh, minty scent, then this will be your oil. Peppermint adds a wonderful aroma to your homemade laundry soap.

5.  **Eucalyptus:** Eucalyptus is a great oil to add to your laundry soap during times of sickness. The oil will freshen clothes and kill germs.

6.  **Lemongrass:** This citrus oil has an earthy smell and makes a great scent, especially for men.

7.  **Roman Chamomile:** Another calming essential oil and great for kids. Roman chamomile adds a beautiful floral scent.

8.  **Cedarwood:** Another one for the men in your life. Cedarwood has a woodsy scent that most men enjoy and has cleansing properties, making it great for your soap.

9.   **Patchouli:** Either you love it or hate it. I am a patchouli lover and am obsessed with the scent. This is another favorite of mine for laundry.

10.  **Jasmine:** If you want to smell like a bed of flowers all day, then add jasmine to your laundry soap. Jasmine is calming and can help with stress and anxious feelings.

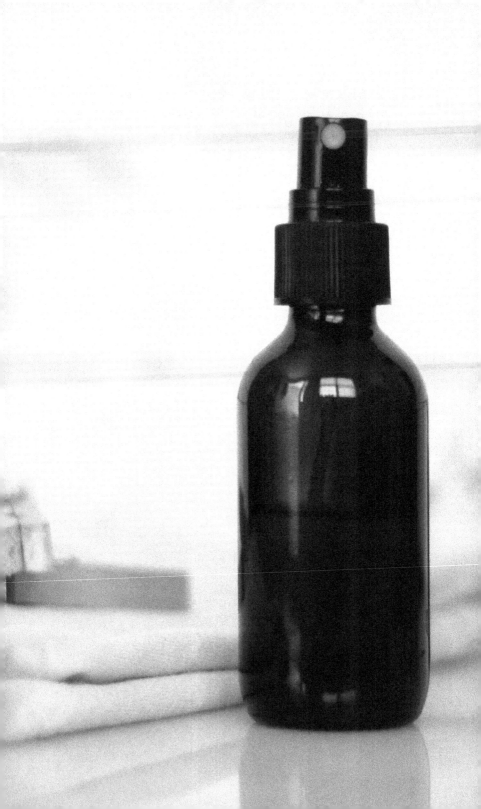

# Spot Treatment

I get asked about spot treatments for laundry all the time. I'll admit that most of the time, I just throw dirty clothes into the machine (not sorted by colors), add some homemade soap, and run it. I am not fancy when it comes to laundry, and I am definitely not particular about clothes. My daughter wears fancy dresses every day, and my boys dress themselves. We don't separate church clothes and play clothes. I just don't care or have the energy to fight about clothes. If they are dressed, I am happy. If you're as busy as I am, I'm sure you feel the same.

With all that being said, sometimes I will have a particular shirt or outfit that I want to keep in good condition for more than one wear. So if I notice a stain, I will spray it first with this spot treatment before washing it. It works great for removing pesky stains!

## Ingredients

+ 1 cup water
+ ⅛ cup castile soap (I use Dr. Bronner's unscented)
+ 2 tablespoons vegetable glycerin
+ 10 drops lemon essential oil
+ Glass spray bottle

## Instructions

1. Add all of the ingredients to a glass spray bottle.

2. Shake until well combined.

## How to Use

1. Spray the spot generously with the spot remover.

2. Message the liquid into the spot.

3. Allow it to sit for about 10 minutes.

4. Wash like normal.

# Fabric Softener

Fabric softener can help eliminate static and wrinkles, soften clothes, and add a beautiful scent to your clothes. I love making my own laundry soap, but when I first made the switch, I missed that classic Tide smell. Adding a fabric softener helped to get that clean scent I was used to.

It is easy to make and use, and it won't leave any chemicals or artificial fragrances on your clothes. It is safe for HE (high efficiency) washing machines and front loaders. This recipe is similar to the dryer sheet recipe, but instead of adding in cloths, you can pour the liquid straight into the washing machine.

You can store this softener in an old fabric softener or laundry detergent container or use a mason jar. I find that old containers work best for pouring the fabric softener into the washing machine.

## Ingredients

+ 1 cup of water
+ 1 cup vinegar
+ 1 tablespoon vegetable glycerin
+ 10–15 drops essential oils

## Instructions

1.  Mix all the ingredients in a mason jar or old laundry soap jug. Shake well to combine.

**Notes**

Add ¼ cup per load. If your washing machine doesn't have a separate compartment for fabric softener, add it to the last rinse cycle. This recipe will keep for 1–2 weeks when stored in an airtight container.

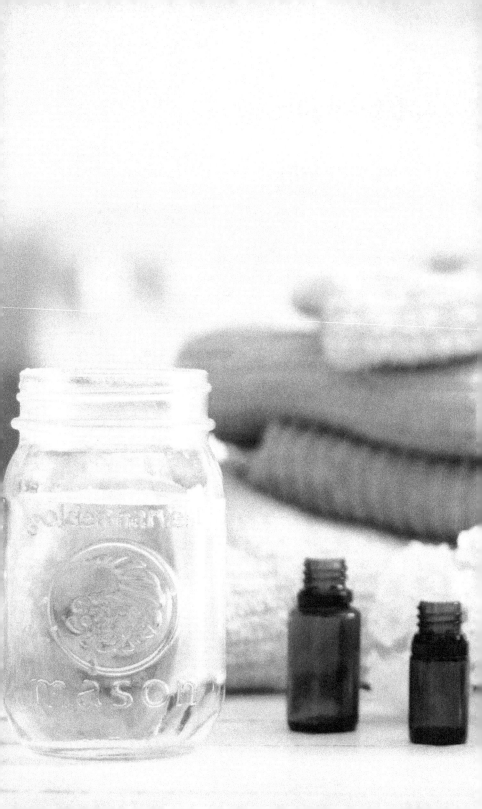

# Natural Bleach

When I first switched to all-natural products in the laundry room, I kept
a bottle of bleach up high on the laundry room shelf. It was my "just in
case I needed it" bottle. Keeping whites white can be hard, especially
with kids. I am happy to say that the "just in case" bleach is no longer in
the laundry room.

I have created a natural solution for whitening my whites. Now that
I have a natural solution, I use it more often, and not just for those
emergencies. Just like all the other recipes in this chapter, making
your own bleach is easy to do, and it can be used just like conventional
bleach. If you're looking for some instant gratification, this is the recipe
to try. You likely already know that store-bought bleach is harmful to
your lungs and known to cause dizziness if inhaled, so the benefits of this
natural product in your home will be immediate.

## Ingredients

+ 1 cup hydrogen peroxide
+ 1 cup baking soda
+ ½ cup lemon juice
+ 15 drops lemon essential oil
+ 8 cups distilled water

## Instructions

1. Mix all the ingredients into a large mason jar or an empty laundry
   soap container.

2. Shake well before each use.

3. Add ½ a cup for a small load and 1 cup for a large load of
   laundry. Pour into the bleach compartment.

## How to Use

If you are dealing with a stubborn stain, you can soak clothes in water
and a cup of bleach overnight before running the load.

### Washer Cleaner

Cleaning your washer might not be on your normal cleaning list or might be something you have never done. It is a once-a-year kind of thing for me, but maybe I should do it more often, given the kind of things that end up in my washer. My kids are either in the woods, covered in mud, sticky, or all of the above at the end of every day. Muddy shoes end up in our washer a lot, too.

This "washer cleaner" is more of a tip than a recipe because it only requires one ingredient: distilled white vinegar! Vinegar is great for cleaning washing machines, and there is no need to add anything else. The process will look a little different depending on how long you've had your machine. Some newer washers even have a clean cycle.

If your washer doesn't have a clean cycle, you can **pour a cup of vinegar** into the detergent compartment and run the longest cycle on hot. Once the load is done, wipe out the seal or any nook or cranny with a warm cloth.

If needed, you can run the washer one more time without anything in it to clean the vinegar smell out.

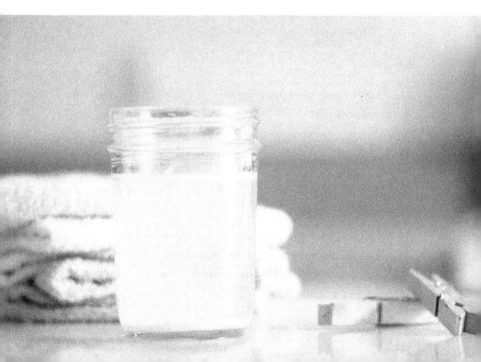

# Dryer Sheets

One of my absolute favorite smells is clean clothes in a dryer. When you're outside near the dryer vent, and you can smell the fresh laundry scent? Oh man, I love that. That particular scent reminds me of being at my grandma's house as a kid.

Once I stopped using conventional laundry detergent, fabric softener, or dryer sheets, that smell became less familiar. However, now that I use essential oils, it is better than ever. When I first started making my own soap, I was lazy and overly frugal and didn't always add essential oils.

The soap still worked great, but I missed that fresh, clean smell. Now, I always add essential oils and, combined with these dryer sheets, and my laundry smells even better. Plus, the dryer sheets work well at softening the clothes.

**Ingredients**

+ 1 cup white vinegar
+ 20–30 drops of essential oils
+ Cotton cloths

**Instructions**

1.  Mix the vinegar and essential oils into a small bowl and stir until well combined.

2.  Cut old cotton t-shirts or fabric remnants into 5-inch squares. You can also use reusable cotton baby wipes.

3.  Fold the fabric pieces to fit inside of a mason jar or other airtight container.

4.  Pour the vinegar and essential oil mixture over the cloth wipes. (I made 12 cloths and used all the liquid. If you make less, you may not need all the liquid. You don't want to saturate them.)

## How to Use

Add 1–2 cloth dryer sheets per load. Before putting the cloths into the dryer, squeeze excess liquid back into the storage container.

**Notes**

These double as a fabric softener and dryer sheet. The vinegar helps to soften clothes and leaves no residue on the laundry. Don't worry; your clothes won't smell vinegary. As the clothes dry, the vinegar smell will diminish. The essential oils will add a beautiful scent to your clothes, and you can customize it to smell however you want. The vinegar and essential oils both help to reduce static.

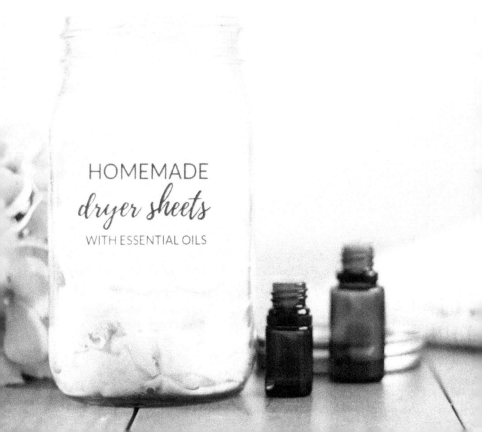

HOMEMADE
*dryer sheets*
WITH ESSENTIAL OILS

# Laundry Scent Boosters

In the eight years I've been making my own laundry products, I have perfected my recipes for laundry powder and homemade dryer sheets. These DIY laundry scent boosters compliment the laundry soap, leaving the clean clothes with a lasting scent. I haven't bought laundry soap since the first time I made it with all-natural products. Now that I am a mother of five doing laundry is a never-ending job.

These homemade laundry scent boosters are just the thing to add to your all-natural laundry products. Just as the name suggests, they boost the scent. Using natural soaps most certainly gets your clothes clean, but if you want that fresh, long-lasting scent that conventional soap leaves behind, then you may want to try this.

**Ingredients**

+ 1 cup of Epsom salt
+ ¼ cup of baking soda
+ 20–30 drops of your preferred essential oil (wild orange and lavender are my favorites)

**Instructions**

1. Mix all the ingredients into a bowl.

2. Whisk together until everything is well combined.

3. Store in an airtight container.

**How to Use**

Simply sprinkle ¼ cup of the "booster" over the clothes before starting the load. Use the normal amount of laundry soap. This recipe is safe to use on HE washers, front loaders, and regular washer machines.

Lavender and wild orange are great for laundry because of their cleansing and purifying properties and their ability to cover the odor. They smell great together, too.

**Notes**

The shelf life is one year. I prefer to make a larger batch at a time and store it in a half-gallon mason jar with a lid. Then I don't have to make it as often. Also, you don't have to use this on every load. I throw it into any load that is extra stinky and dirty. Think workout clothes.

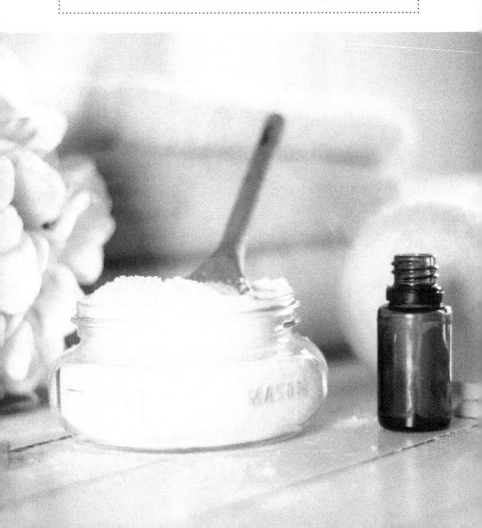

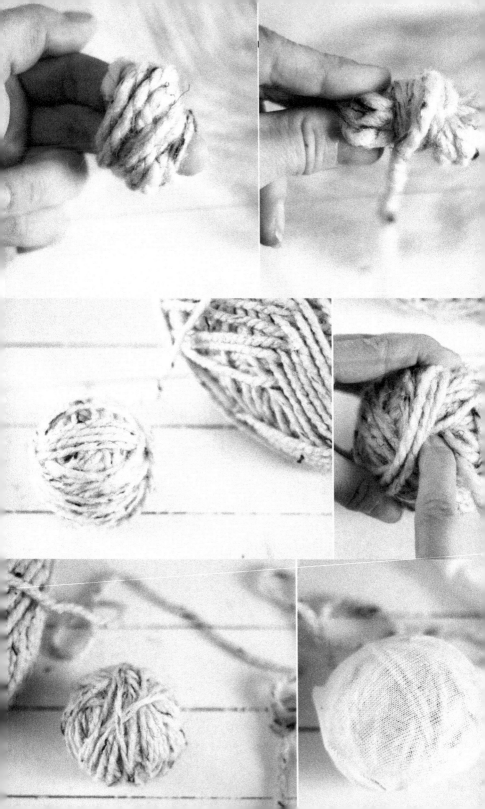

# Dryer Balls

I love using dryer balls. They help make your clothes dry faster and remove static. If you add essential oils to them, which I highly recommend, they will also add an extra scent to your clean clothes. You can buy dryer balls from the store or online, or you can make your own.

Making your own is very simple, and all you need is wool yarn. I am not much of a tailor or seamstress, and even I can make dryer balls; they are that easy.

**Materials**

+ Yarn
+ Essential oils

**Instructions**

1. Start by wrapping the yarn around two fingers. Wrap it one way a few times and then wrap it in another direction, making an X. This will be the center of your dryer ball.

2. Keep wrapping the yarn around the center tightly, forming it into a ball shape. Continue doing this until the ball is about the size of a tennis ball.

3. Once you reach the size you want, you will need to secure the loose piece of string. You can simply tuck it under several under strands. Or you can use a needle or hook to push it in farther.

4. Stick the dryer ball into a nylon stocking or pantyhose. Cut and tie it off on both sides.

5. Wash the dryer ball with a few towels or linens on high heat. This will help to fuse the ball together and make it ready to use.

6. It may take two washes. You can tell it is done when no single thread can be moved around on the outside of the ball. You may even see some fibers coming through the nylon.

7.   Cut the nylon off and remove the dryer ball.

8.   Add 4–6 drops of essential oil on each ball and toss them in the dryer. I leave mine in the dryer and add more essential oils every other week or when I start to notice the clothes aren't smelling like the oils anymore.

## Best Essential Oil Blends for Laundry

The best part about making your own laundry products is choosing the scent. Sometimes, I am simple and go with a single oil, and other times I get a little fancier and use a blend of oils. Lavender and wild orange is my favorite scent combination, and tea tree is the best for covering up that mildew smell.

Over the years, I have tried many blends and haven't found one I didn't like. You can get creative and mix and match however you please. Here are some of my favorites to get you started.

These essential oils are great for laundry because of their cleansing and purifying properties and their ability to cover odor. They smell great together, too.

### My Favorite Blend

Lavender + lemon + wild orange + tea tree

### Citrus

Lemon + wild orange + lime
Wild orange + tangerine + bergamot
Tangerine + lime + grapefruit

### Fresh

Eucalyptus + lavender
Peppermint + wild orange
Siberian fir + Roman chamomile
Cypress + lemon

### Clean

Tea tree + lavender + lemon
Lavender + lemon + peppermint
Rosemary + lemon

### Floral

Lavender + patchouli + wild orange
Roman chamomile + lemon
Geranium + clary sage + ylang-ylang

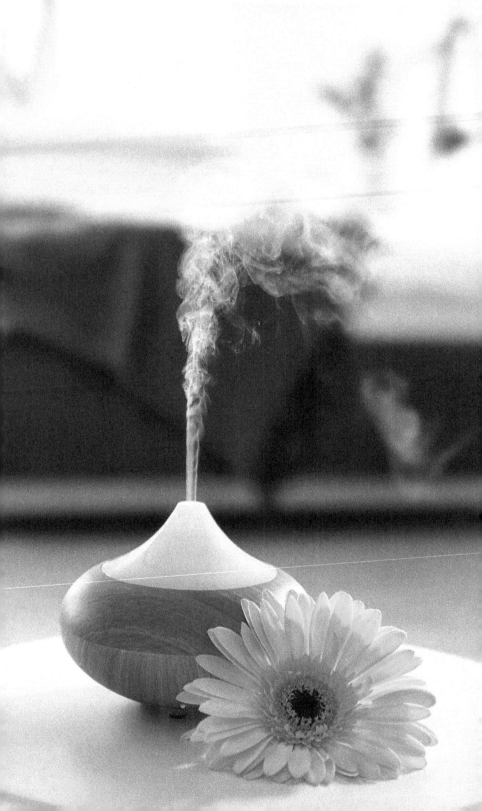

# CHAPTER 4
# Natural Bedroom Remedies

Essential oils can help promote a certain mood, whether it is uplifting or calming. As you breathe in their aroma, molecules travel through the nasal cavity to the part of the brain known as the limbic system. This is the part of the brain that controls emotions, stress responses, and memories. This is why smells can bring back certain memories or be used to help you relax.

In this chapter, you will find calming and relaxing recipes to cozy up the bedroom. From linen sprays to nighttime diffuser blends, these essential oil recipes will help promote a healthy night's rest and make falling asleep even easier. In a house of seven people, anything I can use to make sleep last a little longer or be a little sweeter is a must. Most nights, we have the essential oil diffusers going, and my kids are great little sleepers—whether it is the oils or a blessing, I am not about to fix what isn't broken.

**Simple Tips to Keep the Bedrooms Clean**

My number one tip is to have less stuff. The fewer things in the room, the easier it is to keep clean. I wouldn't call myself a minimalist, but I am close. Each one of my kids only has five play outfits, one nice outfit, pajamas, and, depending on the season, snowsuits or swimsuits in their dressers. I keep it minimal, and it makes the dressers stay cleaner.

I keep bins down low so the kids can put away their toys, shoes, and other belongings by themselves. With less stuff and all storage at their level, it is easier for them to clean their rooms.

I make my bed every single day; in fact, my husband jokes that I would make it with him still in it, as it is the first thing I do. It takes less than two minutes and makes my room instantly look put together.

# Linen Spray

This stuff is my favorite for a couple of reasons. One, I like deliciously-scented linens, and two, I like a good night's sleep. Sleeping is a glorious thing if you sleep soundly. Unfortunately, that isn't the case for many people. Sleep can pose a problem every night and be a struggle in both children and adults.

Some nights, when I lie down to go to sleep, my brain starts going a million miles a minute, thinking of all the things I have to do tomorrow and what I should have done differently that day. Does this happen to anyone else? This linen spray is made with floral essential oils that can help to turn the brain off and promote calmness. Misting your sheets with this spray before bed can make such a difference and help you to drift off into a peaceful sleep.

## Ingredients

+ 4-ounce glass spray bottle
+ 5 drops lavender essential oil
+ 5 drops Roman chamomile essential oil
+ 3 drops vetiver essential oil
+ Witch hazel

## Instructions

1. Add the essential oils to the spray bottle and top off with witch hazel.

2. Shake well before each use.

3. Lightly mist sheets and pillowcases before bed.

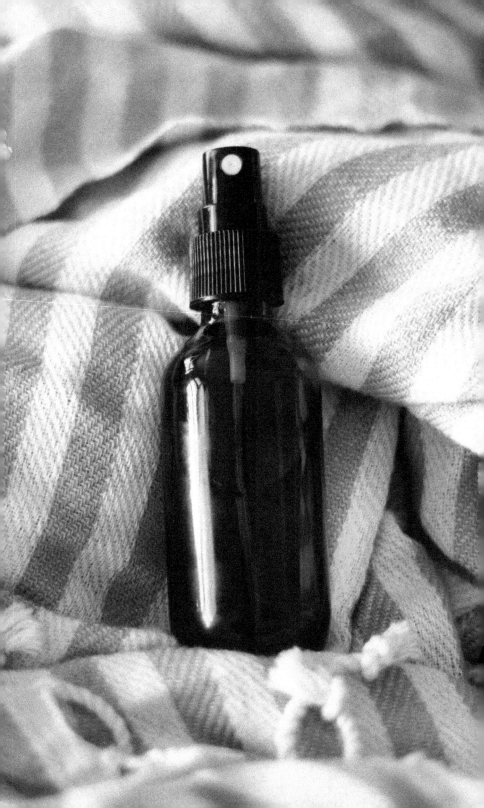

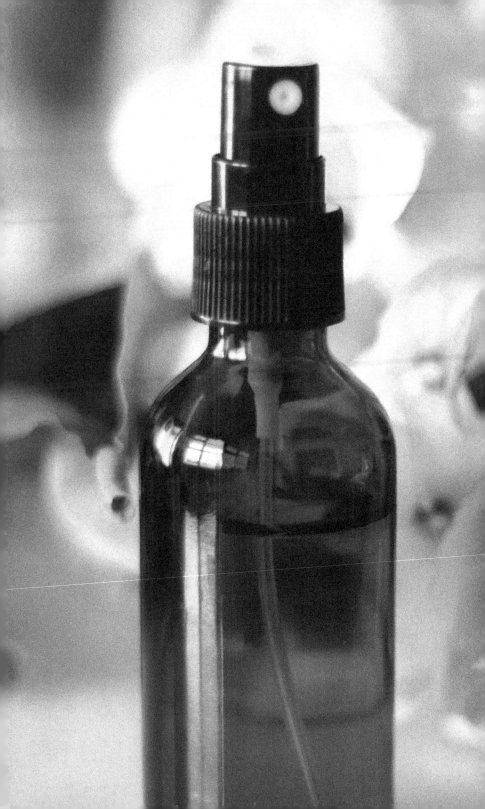

# Air Freshener

This recipe is similar to the linen spray but made with essential oils that are great at deodorizing. I live in a house full of little ones, and though they are cute, they can be stinky. Lots of diapers, socks, spilled milk, and soiled sheets are all part of the whole mom thing.

Having a natural air freshener on hand in each bedroom is a must. We are grabbing for it all the time, and it works to freshen the air and leaves behinds a clean scent. I will share a few different blends of essential oils to try because we love to switch it up over here and have tried quite a few.

## Ingredients

+ 4-ounce glass spray bottle
+ 5 drops lemon essential oil
+ 5 drops lime essential oil
+ 3 drops Siberian fir essential oil
+ Witch hazel

## Instructions

1. Add the essential oils to the spray bottle and top off with witch hazel.

2. Shake well before each use.

3. Mist into the air as needed.

### Other Essential Oil Blends to Try

### Orange Mint

5 drops peppermint
5 drops wild orange

### Zesty Citrus

6 drops bergamot
3 drops ginger
6 drops lime

### Field of Flowers

5 drops lavender
5 drops geranium
5 drops patchouli

### Citrus Bliss

5 drops wild orange
5 drops grapefruit
5 drops lemon

# Furniture Polish

Okay, so have I mentioned my love for cleaning yet? It's weird, but I love to clean. I like a clean house, which helps me keep calm, but I like the chore, too. Dusting is one of those things that needs to be done more than I actually do it, however. Why did no one tell me about the reality of my dark furniture collecting dust endlessly when I picked out my bedroom set?

Since having kids, getting around to deep cleaning and things like dusting has gotten harder to keep up with. I still like a clean home, but, as you probably know, time doesn't always allow me to make it so. So I made up a simple dusting solution that works well to keep furniture dust-free and polished longer. This is a must with kids or hectic schedules. All you need is olive oil and orange essential oil. I use a microfiber cloth to dust and keep it next to the dusting solution under the sink. I recommend you do this too, as it makes it easy to grab and go. The solution will remove dust, polish, and shine.

## Ingredients

+ ½ cup olive oil
+ 10 drops orange essential oil

## Instructions

1. Pour the olive oil into a small mason jar. Add in the drops of essential oils.

2. Secure the lid and stir/shake to mix the oils.

3. Put a quarter-size amount on a microfiber cloth and rub onto wood furniture.

# Massaging Lotion

My husband and I often do in-home date nights. We love to go out, but finding babysitters can be hard, so doing in-home date nights works too. The ideal in-home date night involves the kids going to bed early (a mama can hope, right?), a fancy home-cooked dinner, preferably made by my husband, a massage, and a movie.

I have only had a professional massage once, so I don't have much to compare it to, but I think my husband can do a pretty good massage. For this, using a good lotion is a must. In my recipe, I add soothing and cooling essential oils that help with muscle aches and pains.

**Ingredients**

+ Coconut oil
+ Olive oil
+ Shea butter
+ Cocoa butter
+ Essential oils (I list my favorites below)
+ Mason jars (for storage)

**Instructions**

1. Melt equal parts of each ingredient (besides essential oils) in a double boiler. I make my own double boiler by placing a bowl over a pot of boiling water.

2. After the mixture is melted together, place the bowl in the freezer until it's set up a bit; you should be able to press your thumb into the mixture, and it should hold an indent.

3. Add 20 drops of essential oils.

4. Using a hand mixer or stand-up mixer, whip the ingredients together.

5. Store in an airtight container.

## Best Essential Oils for Massaging Lotion

**Peppermint:** Peppermint has a cooling effect on the body and can relieve tension. Adding peppermint oil to the body butter can make it great for muscle and joint discomfort.

**Cypress:** Cypress oil can calm and relax muscle spasms and works to soothe sore muscles.

**Marjoram:** Marjoram oil can relax muscles by its soothing and calming properties.

**Lavender:** Lavender is my favorite essential oil for calming and relaxing. It helps to calm the body and ease tension.

I add 5 drops each of peppermint, cypress, marjoram, and lavender for my massaging lotion.

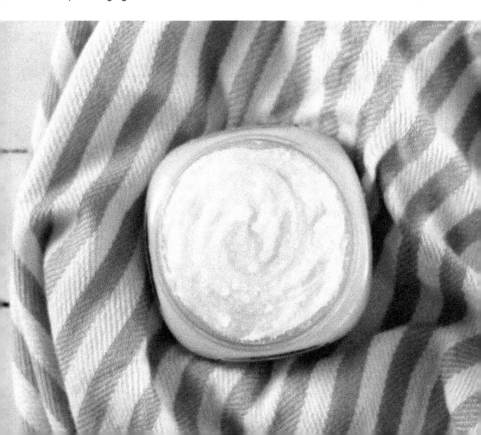

# Rosemary Mint Soy Candle

Making your own candles is much easier than you think. Seriously, anyone can do it. And I am going to teach you the easiest way to do it. The hardest part about candle-making is cleaning the wax out of all the utensils and tools you used to make the candle. So I am going to show you how to do this without using *any* dishes.

Using a crockpot takes all the work out of candle-making and leaves you with nothing to clean up afterward. You can make candles in mason jars, old coffee mugs, antique cups, or crocks. Whatever you have lying around will work.

## Ingredients

+ Soy wax
+ Candle wicks
+ Tape
+ Hole puncher
+ 40 drops rosemary essential oil
+ 40 drops peppermint essential oil
+ Small container or mason jar
+ Crockpot
+ Decorations (optional)

## Instructions

1. Put a couple of cups of water in the bottom of the crockpot and turn it on high heat.

2. Fill the mason jars with soy wax.

3. Place the jars into the crockpot and put the lid on.

4. Allow the wax to melt. You will notice that as the wax melts, it will shrink. You may need to add more wax as it melts.

5.  Once the wax is completely melted, carefully remove the mason jars from the crockpot.

6.  Let them cool slightly, then add in essential oils.

7.  Place the wick in the center of the jar and secure it while the wax dries. The easiest way to keep the wick in the middle of the jar is by placing a piece of tape over the jar and punching a hole in the middle to stick the wick through.

8.  Once the wax is completely hardened, you can trim the wick, and it is ready to light. It should be about a ½-inch long.

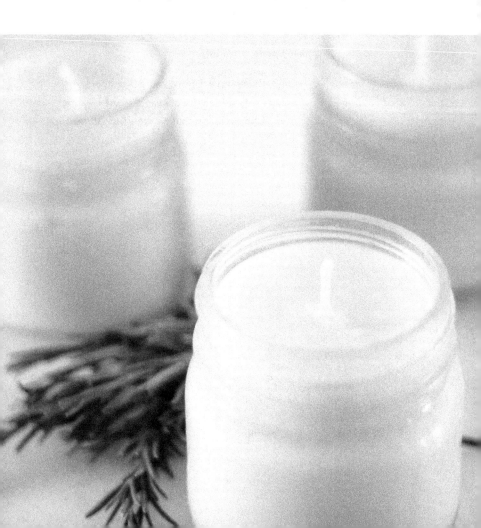

# Roll-On Perfumes

I mostly use my oils for natural remedies, cleaning, and skincare but recently discovered the fun of making perfumes. Most essential oils smell amazing, and combining different ones is a fun way to make an all-natural perfume. Homemade perfumes make beautiful gifts, too.

I like to make perfumes straight in a roller bottle to make them easy to apply. I keep one in my purse so I can freshen up anywhere. I like to add dried flowers to add more scent, and they look so pretty. It is important to make sure the flowers are completely dry before adding them to the oil to keep them from browning. You can purchase dried flowers or dry your own by hanging them upside down for a few days.

The fun of making your own perfume is getting to create a custom scent. You can use single essential oils with added dried flowers or use a blend of oils. I will share some of my favorite scents, but be creative and try some of your own, too.

You will need a carrier oil for this recipe, and it is important to use one with little to no scent. My favorite is fractionated coconut oil.

## Ingredients

+ 10 mL roller bottle (If adding dried flowers, use clear glass rollers so you can see them.)
+ 15–20 drops of essential oils
+ Dried flowers
+ Carrier oil

## Instructions

1. Place dried flowers or buds into a roller bottle. Fill it about halfway.

2. Add in a carrier oil, leaving a little room at the top for the essential oils.

3.  Drop in essential oils.

4.  Secure roller ball top and flip back upside down a few times to mix oils.

5.  Roll on neck, wrists, and chest as needed.

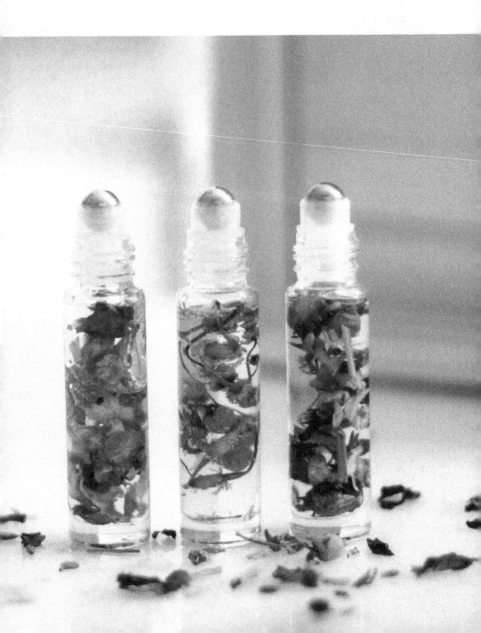

## Perfume Blends

### Citrus Spice

5 drops tangerine essential oil
5 drops lemon essential oil
3 drops ginger essential oil
3 drops pink pepper essential oil

### Floral

5 drops rose essential oil
5 drops jasmine essential oil
3 drops wild orange essential oil
3 drops ylang-ylang essential oil

### Bright and Cheery

5 drops grapefruit essential oil
5 drops wild orange essential oil
5 drops lemon essential oil
3 drops spearmint essential oil

### Calming and Relaxing

5 drops Roman chamomile essential oil
5 drops lavender essential oil
3 drops bergamot essential oil
3 drops sandalwood essential oil

## Best Essential Oils for Sleep

When I first bought essential oils, I used them more during the day than overnight. Once I started having kids, it flipped. Getting a good night's sleep is so important as a mom and for kids. I love making roller bottles and diffuser blends to promote a healthy night's sleep. Not only does the relaxing smell of lavender help me to fall asleep faster, but it can also help me to sleep longer. I diffuse essential oils overnight for my kids, too.

Most people know lavender can help with calming and relaxing, but it isn't the only oil we use at night. In fact, several essential oils can be used to help turn the brain off and make you drift off into a peaceful night's sleep. Like most things, you can use a single oil or a blend of oils. Everyone is different, and certain essential oils may help one person sleep better than others. It is important to try a few different essential oils and blends to see what works best for you.

### Sleep Diffuser Blends

3 drops lavender
3 drops Roman chamomile
3 drops vetiver

3 drops ylang-ylang
3 drops wild orange
3 drops copaiba

3 drops cedarwood
3 drops sandalwood
3 drops lavender

### Sleep Roller Bottles

5 drops lavender
5 drops vetiver
5 drops Roman chamomile
5 drops frankincense

5 drops copaiba
5 drops jasmine
3 drops wild orange
3 drops bergamot

10 drops frankincense
10 drops lavender

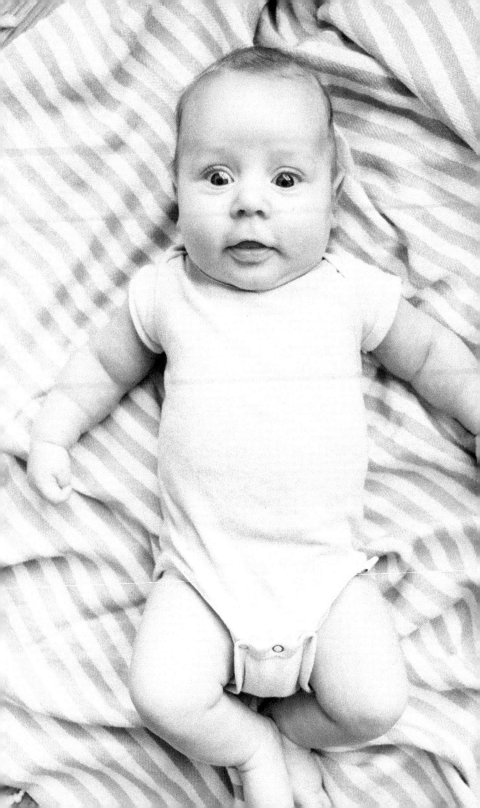

# CHAPTER 5

# Natural Baby and Kids Remedies

All parents will understand that when your first baby is born, your perspective changes. My daughter was so tiny and perfect, and, as a new mom, I was worried about everything. I thought about her first cold, her first fall, and all the what-ifs.

A baby's skin is so smooth and delicate, I worried about any creams, ointments, or soap I put on her. I quickly realized that making my own baby products would be the best option. Yes, you can buy safe products from the store, but not without spending an arm and a leg. I found that making my own was much more cost-effective and the products worked just as well.

In this chapter, I will teach you how to make everything you need, from the products used for bathing your children to boost their immune systems. Being a mom can be hard, but having a few natural remedies on hand will come in handy.

# Diaper Cream

Every parent needs to have this diaper cream—it is that good. If you have ever had a baby, you know that diaper rash is just one of the things you will have to deal with. Some babies get it worse than others, but I have never had one that has escaped it altogether.

This cream works so well, and it is great for sensitive skin. I make it with cocoa butter, coconut oil, zinc oxide, bentonite clay, and tea tree essential oil. Cocoa butter and coconut oil are moisturizing and can help to soothe sore skin. Zinc oxide is commonly found in conventional diaper creams and sunscreen; this is why sometimes I will use my homemade sunscreen for diaper rashes if I don't have any diaper cream whipped up already.

The zinc oxide creates a moisturizing barrier to help keep the skin dry. Bentonite clay is rich in many vital nutrients, including calcium, magnesium, silica, sodium, potassium, and iron. It has amazing benefits for the skin. I add tea tree oil for its antifungal properties. Does your baby have a rash that no diaper cream can shake? It could be because your baby has a yeast infection. The added tea tree can help with that.

To make this diaper cream, you will need a double boiler, wooden spoon, mixing bowl, and a mason jar with a lid.

## Ingredients

+ ¼ cup cocoa butter
+ 1 tablespoon coconut oil
+ 1 tablespoon bentonite clay
+ 1 tablespoon zinc oxide
+ 2 drops tea tree essential oil

## Instructions

1. Place the cocoa butter and coconut oil in a double boiler. Melt over medium heat, stirring occasionally.

2.  Remove from the heat and add in the clay, zinc oxide, and tea tree essential oil.

3.  Pour into a mason jar with an airtight lid.

---

**Notes**

It is important to use glass and wooden appliances when working with clay. I use a glass bowl for my ingredients and stir with a wooden spoon.

---

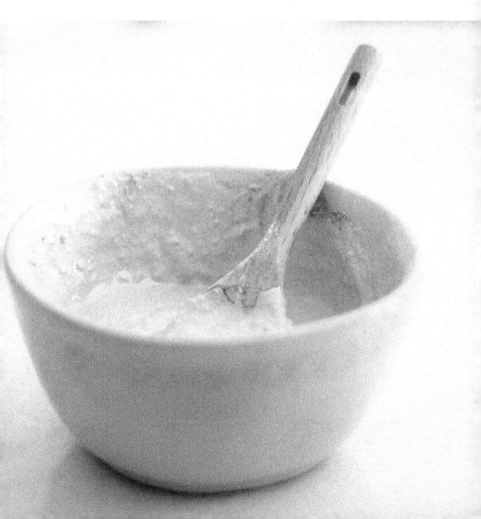

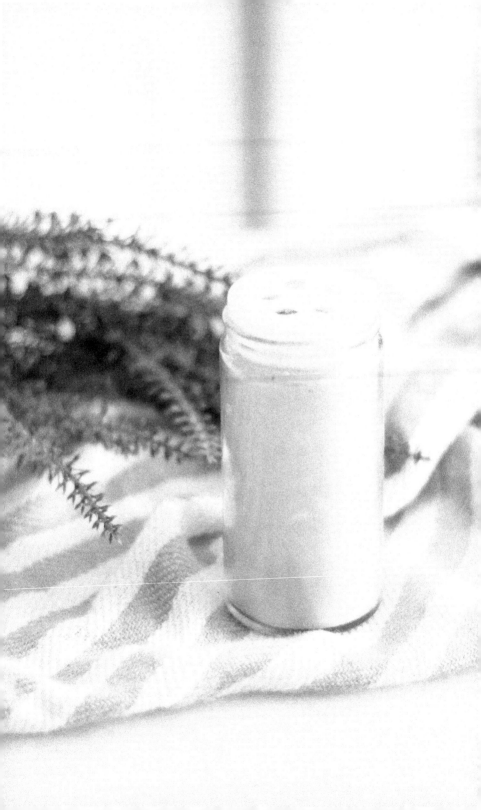

# Baby Powder

I am one of four girls and am second in the lineup. As my sister mentioned at the beginning of the book, I have always been obsessed with babies and remember helping with my little sisters a lot. I am not sure if my mom would call it helping, but hey, this is my book and my memories. We used baby powder at most diaper changes. It was a must-have product back then, but now, not so much. Many studies have come out since then out about the dangers of talc found in most baby powders and how it can lead to serious respiratory illnesses. Baby powder came to a halting stop for a while, but it seems it is coming back now that we know what not to add.

Thankfully, making your own is so simple and is much healthier for your baby. In fact, you only need two ingredients to make an effective baby powder. Baby powder helps to keep your baby's bottom dry, preventing diaper rash.

## Ingredients

+ ⅛ cup arrowroot powder
+ ⅛ cup bentonite clay
+ 3–5 drops lavender essential oil (optional)
+ Storage container (old spice containers make great vessels for baby powder)
+ Wooden spoon
+ Small mixing bowl

## Instructions

1. Add arrowroot powder and clay into a small glass bowl.

2. Drop in essential oil.

3. Using a wooded spoon, stir until everything is well combined.

4. Pour mixture into a storage container. Glass storage is best for clay and essential oils.

# Reusable Wipes and Spray Solution

If you are already using cloth diapers, adding in cloth wipes is a no-brainer. I have used cloth with all my kids and love how much money it saves! Of course, it is better for the environment, too. I started building up my stash of cloth diapers when I was pregnant with my first and used those same diapers for all my kids. Talk about cost-effective.

I have made homemade baby wipes with paper towels and a solution, bought natural wipes, and dabbled in using cloth. I found that using cloth wipes with a little homemade spray was the best solution, especially when we were at home. The solution is easy to make and made with all-natural ingredients, making it safe for babies' sensitive skin.

### Ingredients

+ 4-ounce glass spray bottle
+ 1 teaspoon vitamin E oil
+ 2 drops tea tree oil
+ 2 drops lavender oil
+ Witch hazel

### Instructions

1. Add vitamin E oil and essential oils to the glass spray bottle.

2. Top off with witch hazel.

3. Secure lid and shake well.

### How to Use

Spray the solution straight on the baby's skin or on a clean cloth wipe. Gently wipe the baby's skin clean with wipe.

**Notes**

We keep a wastebasket that has a lid in the bathroom for cloth diapers and wipes. After you use the wipe, just toss it into the wastebasket with the diapers. I wash every four days with my homemade laundry soap. For odor control, add a few drops of lemon essential oil to the bottom of your wastebasket.

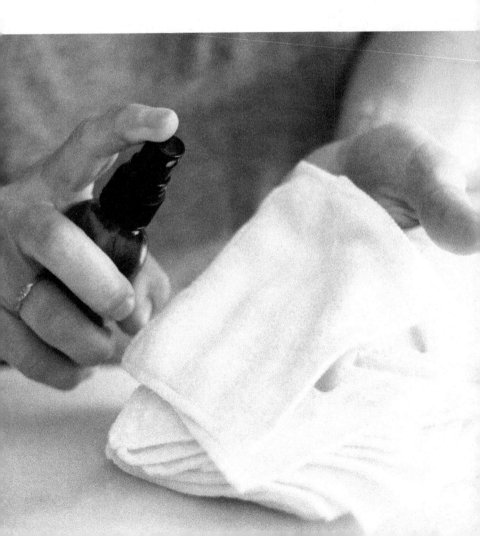

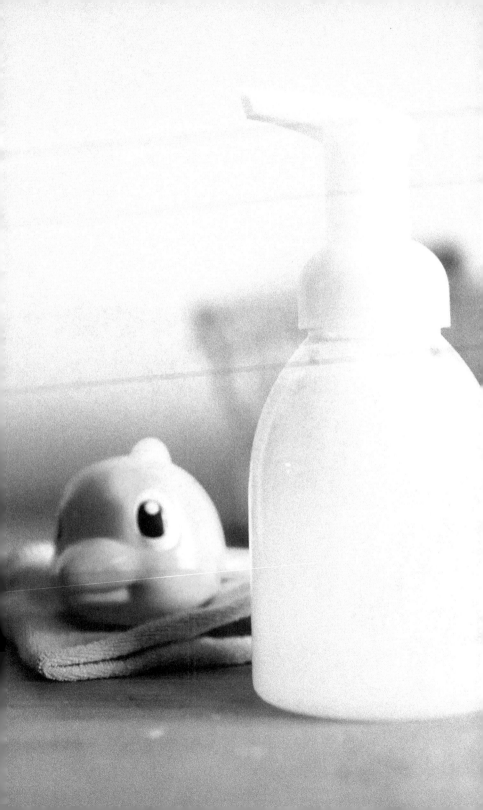

# Baby Wash

Baby skin is delicate and soft; therefore, using a gentle bath wash is important. You can buy natural options, but I found that making my own is cheaper and it is simple to make.

With a few ingredients, you can whip up this baby wash in just a couple of minutes. We have been using this for our children for over a year, and it works well on their skin and hair.

I call it baby wash, but honestly, it works well for older kids, too. My oldest is seven, and she still uses this.

## Ingredients

+ ¼ cup castile soap (I use Dr. Bronner's unscented castile soap)
+ 1 tablespoon glycerin
+ 1 teaspoon fractionated coconut oil
+ 1 teaspoon vitamin E oil
+ 5 drops lavender essential oil
+ 3 drops Roman chamomile essential oil
+ 10-ounce foaming soap container

## Instructions

1. Add all the ingredients to the foaming soap container and top off with water.

2. Shake before each use to combine the ingredients.

# Baby Lotion

Just like the gentle baby wash, using natural baby lotion is a must, too. Baby skin can dry out pretty easily, especially during the winter months from bathing or if they struggle with eczema. If your baby has dry skin, you can apply this baby lotion to keep it moisturized and smooth.

I love to add a little lavender essential oil to my homemade baby products because it is a calming scent and can help promote a better night's sleep. Lavender essential oil is also good for the skin and can help with most skin imperfections, blemishes, and rashes. You will also find vitamin E oil in this lotion. Vitamin E oil is high in antioxidants and works well for treating dry, chapped skin.

### Ingredients

+ 4 tablespoons cocoa butter
+ 4 tablespoons coconut oil
+ 5 drops vitamin E oil
+ 2 drops lavender essential oil
+ Glass mason jar for storage (I prefer using a wide mouth mason jar to make it easier to get the lotion out.)

### Instructions

1. Melt cocoa butter and coconut oil in a double boiler.
2. Once ingredients are melted, remove from heat and allow the mixture to cool slightly.
3. Add in vitamin E oil and lavender essential oil.
4. Store in a glass mason jar with an airtight lid.

### Notes

If you want to whip the lotion to give it a fluffy texture, you can place the bowl in the refrigerator to allow it to set. You want the mixture to hold shape when you press your thumb into it but not solid. Once it is set, you can whip it with a hand mixer or immersion blender.

You can substitute the cocoa butter for shea butter or mango butter.

## Cradle Cap Remedy

Cradle cap is a white or yellow scaly rash common in infants. It is usually harmless and doesn't need medical attention. It can be annoying, look gross, and be tempting to pick off. However, I have read it is best not to pick at it, and picking it off can irritate a baby's scalp. All of my kids had cradle cap to some degree.

I have found that using **coconut oil and a fine-tooth comb** is the best way to remove it. Put a generous about of coconut oil on your baby's head and massage it in. Let it sit for a couple of hours; letting it sit makes it easier to remove. I always did this a couple of hours before I was planning on giving my baby a bath. I just rubbed it in and let them play like normal. After a couple of hours, put the baby in the tub and gently comb the hair with a fine-tooth comb. The cradle cap comes right off like magic!

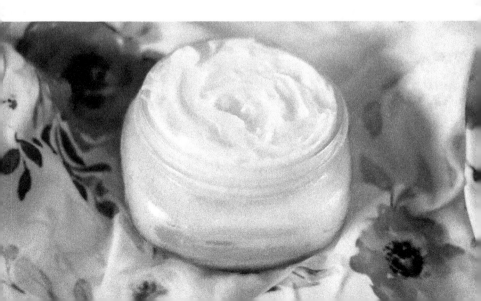

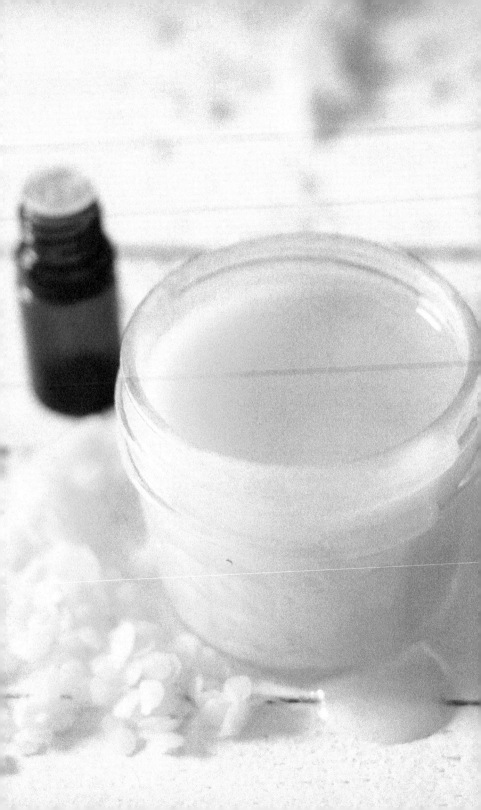

# Natural Coconut Oil Rub

I have several memories of my mom and my babysitter (I had the same sitter from six weeks old until I went to school) rubbing gooey stuff that had a strong scent all over my feet and then covering it up with socks. It wasn't until much later in my life that I found out that stuff had a name, Vicks VapoRub!

As soon as my little one had her first cough, I remembered the Vicks. However, when I went to the store to buy it, I wasn't overly impressed with the ingredients. It has petrolatum in it, which is one of those things I try to avoid. *What can I use instead of Vicks VapoRub?* I wondered. *Could I make my own?*

I found a few recipes online, but of course, I didn't have everything I needed. So in true Laura fashion, I mixed and matched recipes and came up with something that used what I had on hand. And guess what? It worked.

I have added a few more children to the mix since then, and I can't even count how many times I've had to mix up this concoction.

## Ingredients

+ ¼ cup coconut oil
+ ¼ cup cocoa butter
+ 2 tablespoons beeswax
+ 10 drops eucalyptus essential oil
+ 10 drops peppermint essential oil
+ 10 drops lemon essential oil
+ 10 drops clove essential oil

## Instructions

1. Place all the ingredients, except the essential oils, in a double boiler.

2.  Remove from the heat once everything is melted.

3.  Allow to cool slightly, and then add in essential oils.

4.  Store in an airtight glass container.

**Notes**

If making this recipe for children under thirteen, use 5 drops of each essential oil. If making for a baby under the age of one, only use 2 drops of each essential oil.

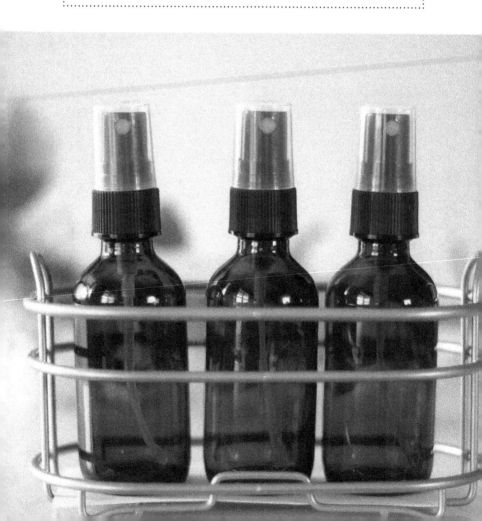

# Essential Oil Sprays for Kids

I love creating room sprays, linen spray, and air fresheners with my essential oils. I love the smell of conventional air refreshers, but I hate spraying chemicals into the air. In my opinion, it seems to defeat the purpose—just me?

I keep a little caddy of room sprays in my kids' room, just for them. These sprays can help freshen the room, promote calmness, and purify the air. As a mama of five, I know these sprays are must-haves for my littles' room. Room sprays are easy to make and easy to use; the kids can even help you with this DIY. Plus, this little set of sprays would make a perfect baby shower gift.

### Kids Air Freshener

3 drops wild orange
2 drops lavender
1 drop bergamot

### Kids Purify the Air

3 drops lemon
2 drops rosemary
1 drop grapefruit

### Kids Pillow and Linen Spray

3 drops lavender
2 drops chamomile
1 drop vetiver

---

**Kids Room Spray**

**Materials**

+ 4-ounce glass spray bottle
+ Essential oils
+ Witch hazel

**Instructions**

1. Drop essential oils into a glass spray bottle.
2. Fill the rest of the bottle with witch hazel. I use unscented.
3. Shake well before each use. Mist spray into the air as needed.

---

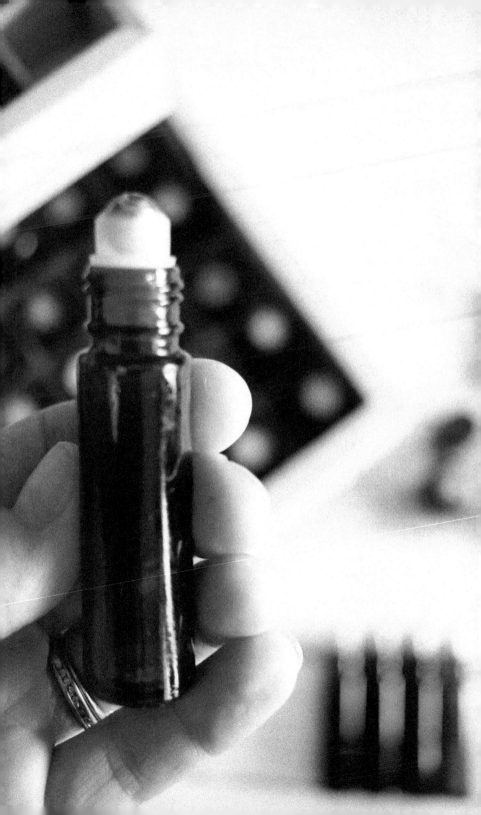

# Essential Oil Roller Bottles for Kids

As a mama, I couldn't imagine life without my essential oils. We go to them often throughout the day, and most often, we are grabbing a roller bottle. Anytime you are using essential oils topically on kids, it is extremely important to dilute them first. My favorite way to dilute essential oils for my kids is by making roller bottles.

Roller bottles make it easy to apply, and the kids can even apply them by themselves. The best place to apply them is on the bottom of the feet, down the spine, or area of concern. Avoid putting essential oils into the ears and eyes.

## Tummy Tamer

3 drops peppermint
2 drops ginger
2 drops fennel
2 drops frankincense
1 drop lemon

## Nightmares

10 drops lavender
10 drops myrrh
6 drops lemon

## Teething Baby

3 drops lavender
3 drops frankincense
3 drops Roman chamomile

## Owie Blend

4 drops tea tree (melaleuca)
4 drops lavender
4 drops frankincense

## Tantrum Tamer

3 drops frankincense
3 drops lavender
2 drops wild orange
2 drops vetiver

## Immune Support

4 drops frankincense
3 drops rose
2 drops wild orange
1 drop oregano

## Sleep Tight

4 drops lavender
3 drops Roman chamomile
2 drops cedarwood
1 drop vetiver

## Good Mood

4 drops wild orange
3 drops sandalwood
2 drops bergamot
1 drop lavender

## Diffuser Blends for Kids

Diffusing essential oils can benefit a child's emotions, mood, and wellness. I have a diffuser in each of my kid's room, and they love to help fill it each day and night. This is a great way to get your kids involved and teach them about natural solutions at a young age. I keep a few of our favorite oils right in their room to make filling them even easier. If you do this, be sure to keep them up high and out of reach of your children.

A few of our favorite blends are for promoting a good night's sleep, boost the immune system, and promoting positive feelings.

### Good Night

3 drops lavender
2 drops copaiba
1 drop Roman chamomile

### Immune Support

2 drops wild orange
2 drops frankincense
2 drop clove

### Happy Day

2 drops wild orange
2 drops bergamot
1 drop lavender
1 drop lemon

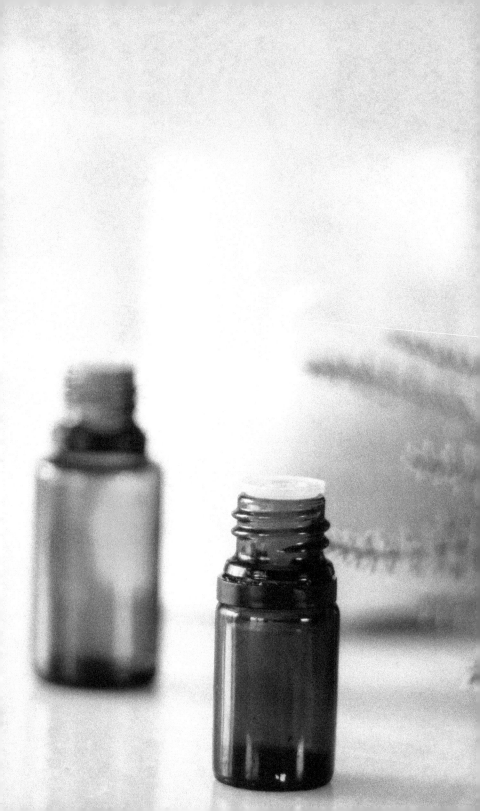

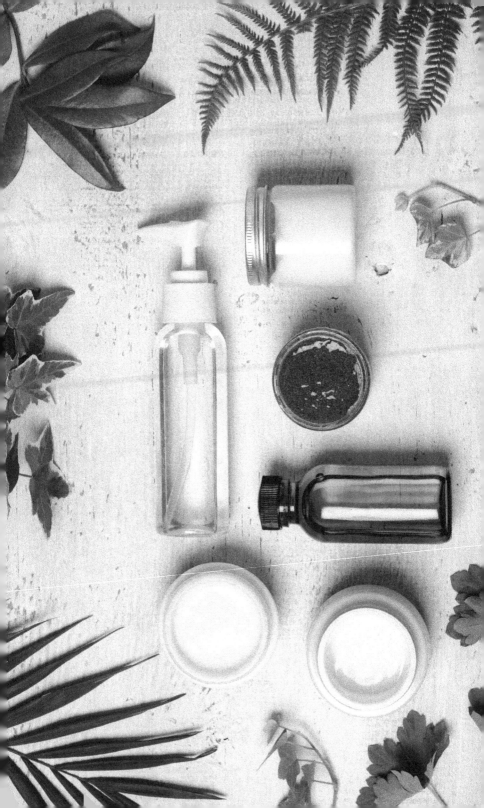

# CHAPTER 6

# Natural Bath and Beauty Remedies

ls, I have transformed my bath and beauty routine to homemade—one thing at a time, of course. If you are looking for "clean beauty" products, you are in the right place, my friends. The amount of chemicals lurking in bath and beauty products is just crazy. It seems harmless to buy the pretty pink bath bombs with sparkles, right? However, the skin is the largest organ of the body, and it absorbs what we put on it like a sponge. This means that pretty bath bomb is being absorbed into the bloodstream.

We know we can't be perfect all of the time and are exposed to toxins daily, but we can do our best to eliminate them within our home. Starting with what we put on our skin and hair can cut that number down.

In this chapter, you will find homemade bath and beauty products that are easy to use and make. I like to keep it simple around here.

# Essential Oil Blends for Bath and Beauty Products

Once you start getting familiar with essential oils, you'll start to note some of your favorite scents. However, if you need a little inspiration, try some of these blends for your bath and beauty products, depending on your mood.

## Citrus

Lemon
Grapefruit
Lime

## Floral

Lavender
Patchouli
Roman chamomile

## Fresh

Lemon
Rosemary
Cypress

## Minty

Spearmint (or peppermint)
Eucalyptus
Wintergreen

## Calming and Relaxing

Lavender
Roman Chamomile
Clary Sage
Lavender
Frankincense
Sandalwood

## Soothing Massage Blend

Peppermint
Eucalyptus
Siberian fir

## Earthy

Sandalwood
Cedarwood
Bergamot

## Best Blend for Women

Lavender
Jasmine
Wild orange
Patchouli

## Best Blend for Men

Cedarwood
Lemongrass
Bergamot

## Best Blend for Children

Lavender
Roman chamomile
Frankincense

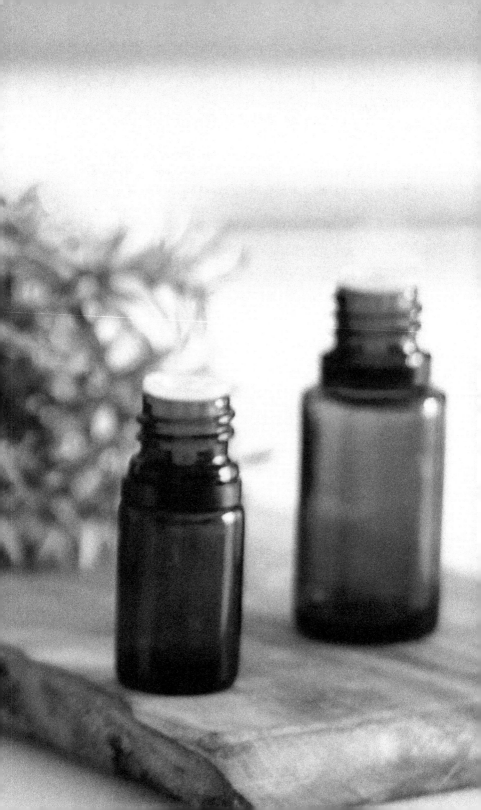

# Calming Bath Soak

Sometimes, at the end of the day, we just need a calming bath—anyone with me? As a mom of five, taking a bath doesn't happen nearly as often as I dream about it, but when it does happen, I make it count. Why get in the tub without some type of soak? I keep a mason jar of this homemade bath soak next to the tub just in case I find the time to hop in.

It is made with Epsom salt, pink Himalayan salt, lavender buds, and my all-time favorite calming essential oils. Not only does it help eliminate the stress of the day, but it also has benefits for the skin and will help you sleep better at night.

## Ingredients

+ 3 cups Epsom salt
+ 1 cup pink Himalayan salt (I prefer using coarse pink Himalayan salt)
+ ¼ cup dried lavender buds
+ 25 drops essential oils (lavender and wild orange are my favorites)

## Instructions

1. In a large bowl, combine the salts.

2. Drop in the essential oils and stir to combine into the salts.

3. Sprinkle in the lavender buds. Toss to combine.

4. Store in an airtight container.

## How to Use

Dissolve ½ of a cup into warm water. For best results, soak for at least 20 minutes.

**Notes**

Salts can harden over time, so be sure you store these in an airtight container. When they do harden, you can break it apart by fluffing it with a fork.

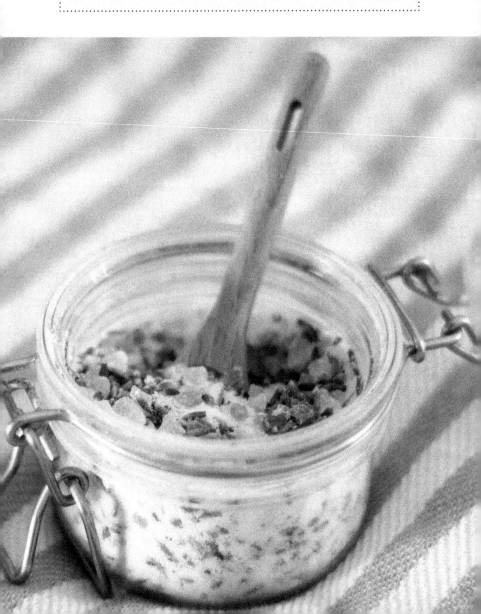

# Muscle Relaxing Bath Salts

Like the calming bath soak, you will need Epsom salt and essential oils for this recipe. Several essential oils can be used for tension and soothing muscles. This bath soak can be used pre- or post-workout, after a long day of work, or if you are experiencing body tension.

Epsom salt can reduce pain and inflammation, reduce stress, and increase magnesium levels.

**Best Essential Oils for Muscle Tension**

**Peppermint:** Peppermint can have a cooling effect on the body and can help to soothe sore muscles.

**Copaiba:** Copaiba can reduce pain due to inflammation.

**Lavender:** Lavender can be used to calm and relax muscles.

**Eucalyptus:** Eucalyptus has a cooling effect on the body and can help reduce inflammation.

**Marjoram:** Marjoram can reduce muscle spasms, nerve discomfort and relax muscles.

I suggest using a combination of all of these oils, but if you don't have them all, you can pick a couple off of this list to add to your bath soak.

## Ingredients

+ 3 cups Epsom salt
+ 20 drops essential oils (choose from the list above)

## Instructions

1. Pour the Epsom salt into a large bowl.
2. Drop in the essential oils and stir to combine into the salt.
3. Store in an airtight container.

## How to Use

Dissolve ½ of a cup into warm water. For best results, soak for at least 20 minutes.

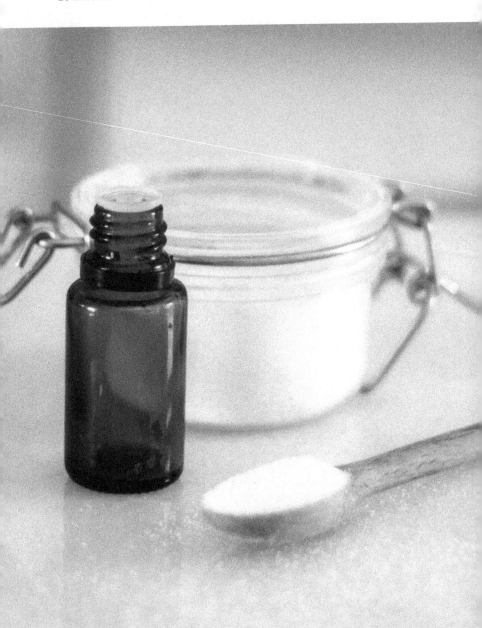

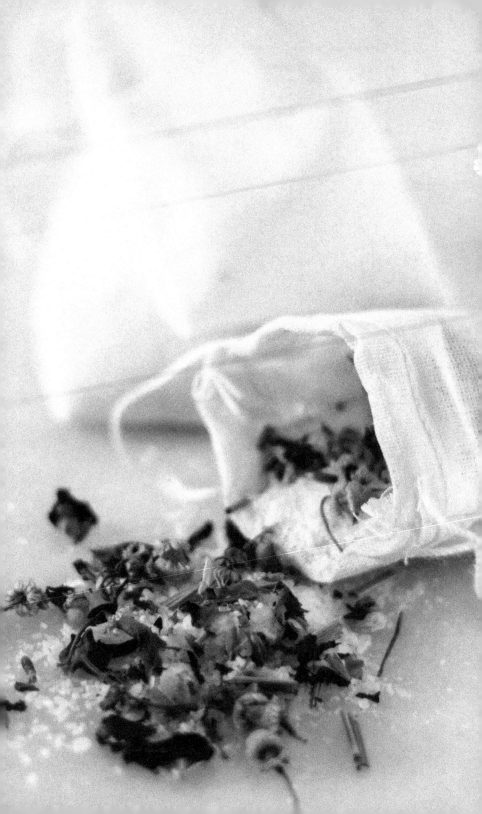

# Bedtime Tub Tea

Slipping into a warm bath with relaxing herbs and oils before bedtime can be one of the best ways to calm down after a busy day. Not only for the body but also the mind. My mind can go in a million different directions when I lie down—instead of going to sleep, I start thinking about all the things on my to-do list tomorrow. I know I'm not alone here.

Certain essential oils can help to turn the brain off and calm the nervous system—something this mom needs before drifting off to sleep. This sleepy time tub tea is just the thing. You can thank me later.

These little tub teas make the perfect gift, too. You can switch up the dried flowers and essential oils you use. Below is my favorite blend.

**Ingredients**

+ 1 cup Epsom salt
+ 1 tablespoon dried lavender
+ 1 tablespoon dried chamomile
+ 1 tablespoon dried rose petals
+ 10 drops lavender essential oil
+ 5 drops jasmine essential oil
+ Muslin tea bags

**Instructions**

1. Pour all the ingredients into a bowl. Stir until everything is combined.

2. Put the mixture in muslin tea bags and tie a knot.

**How to Use**

Fill the bathtub with warm water and swirl the tea bag into the water. Allow it to steep for 10 minutes. Hop in and enjoy.

# Lemon Bath Bombs

We are pretty obsessed with bath bombs over here. They are fun to make and fun to use—what is not to love? My kids beg to take "bath bomb" baths all the time, and everyone loves to pick their scents. We have made a lot of different kinds, but lemon is one of our favorites.

Lemon essential oil is so refreshing, cleansing, and can give you a natural energy boost. Sometimes we leave our bath bombs their natural white color, but my kids prefer to color them. I found some skin-safe natural dye and use it in a lot of my DIYs. It works perfectly to add a little color to our bath bombs.

The first time I made bath bombs, I was shocked at how easy they were to make. I wish I would have tried making them much sooner before buying so many for way too much money at farmer's markets and fairs. Plus, when you make your own, you can customize them however you want.

## Ingredients

+ 1 cup baking soda
+ ½ cup citric acid
+ ½ cup cornstarch
+ ¼ cup Epsom salt
+ ¼ cup melted coconut oil
+ 15–20 drops lemon essential oil
+ Natural yellow dye (optional)
+ Water
+ Spray bottle
+ Bath bomb molds

## Instructions

1. Mix all the dry ingredients in a medium-size bowl. Stir until well incorporated.

2.  Add in the coconut oil, essential oils, and food coloring if using. Whisk together until well combined.

3.  With a spray bottle, spray the mixture with water until the ingredients hold together when squeezed in your hands. Only do one spray at a time. We do not want to over saturate it.

4.  Prepare your bath bomb molds by greasing them with coconut oil. I use these molds, but you can also use a plastic Easter egg or a Christmas ornament.

5.  Press the mixture into both sides of the bath bomb molds and then put the two sides together. Rub the excess mixture off the sides and set aside.

6.  Allow the molds to sit for 24–48 hours or until completely dry and then pop out of the molds.

# Honey and Oatmeal Soap Bar

As much as I am a DIYer, I like to keep it simple—like, really simple. I love making my own soap, even though I cheat by using a melt-and-pour soap base. I would love to make cold-pressed soap bars someday, but for now, melt and pour soap it is. Cold-pressed is a much harder process and requires many more ingredients, whereas anyone can make a melt-and-pour soap bar, even my seven-year-old.

I love that melt-and-pour soap bars are so easy to make, and you can still customize them. You can choose what kind of soap base you want to use, what scent you want to make, and choose what you want to add in. I love adding in oatmeal or coffee to exfoliate the skin.

Oatmeal has so many great benefits for the skin and can help with many skin irritations. You can use quick oats, colloidal oatmeal, or powder oatmeal. You can make your own powder oatmeal by blending oatmeal in a high-speed blender.

Adding in honey gives this soap antiviral and antibacterial properties. Honey is great for natural skincare and will help to keep skin smooth and moisturized as well.

### Ingredients

+ 1 pound shea butter soap base
+ ¼ cup oatmeal (I use regular rolled oats and blend them in my blender to make them finer.)
+ 2 teaspoons honey
+ 40 drops lavender essential oil
+ Silicone soap mold

### Instructions

1. Cut the shea butter soap base into small chunks and place them into a double boiler.

2.   Melt over medium heat. Stir occasionally with a wooden spoon.

3.   Remove from heat when it is completely melted.

4.   Add in oatmeal, honey, and lavender essential oil. Stir to mix.

5.   Pour into a soap mold.

6.   Allow it to completely harden and then pop the soap out of the mold.

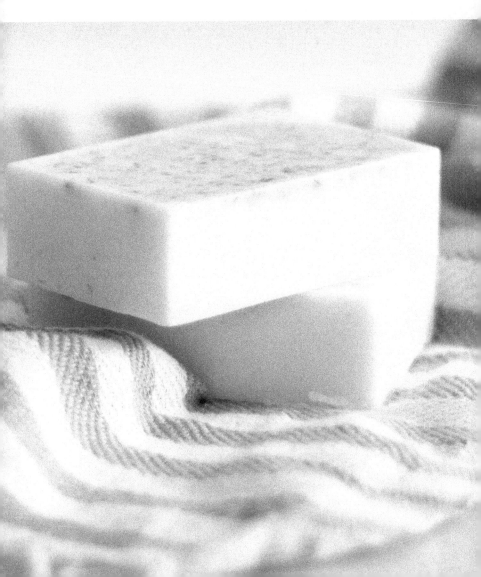

# Natural Hairspray

Y'all know my love for DIYing around here. I love making all different recipes, but hair products are top on my list. I am a simple gal when it comes to hair care, and as long as I have a good stock of dry shampoo, I am good. But after getting so many requests for DIY natural hairspray, I decided to give it a whirl.

I was so happy with how it turned out (and smelled!) that I had to add it to the book. DIY natural hairspray is so easy to make, and you will never guess what ingredient makes it hold your hairstyle. Sugar! Yep, regular white sugar.

So why not just use a store-bought hairspray? As with most things, conventional hairspray is full of chemicals that you shouldn't breathe in and most certainly not spray on your head. Hairsprays can irritate the eyes, nose, throat, skin, and lungs when inhaled.

Switching to homemade hairspray is a much safer option, especially if you are working on getting toxins out of your home. Most hairsprays will have polymers in them, including polyvinylpyrrolidone (PVP), vegetable gums, and gum arabic. You will also find hydrocarbons, propylene glycol, isobutane, propane, and fragrances on the long list of ingredients.

Were you shocked to hear sugar would be in a hair product? Even though sugar isn't something you would want to put in your body, believe it or not, it has benefits for your hair. And your skin. Sugar works well at exfoliating the skin, and it can do the same for your scalp.

Sugar will be the key ingredient in the hairspray and help your hair hold the style you are going for. White sugar is a must, as brown sugar, coconut sugar, honey, and other natural sugars will not work in this recipe.

## Ingredients

+ 1 cup water
+ 1.5 tablespoons white sugar
+ 1 tablespoon high proof alcohol (vodka, rum, or gin will work)
+ 5 drops rosemary essential oil
+ 5 drops lavender essential oil
+ Glass spray bottle

## Instructions

1. Bring the water to a boil over high heat and then add in the sugar.

2. Stir the sugar water until all the sugar is dissolved.

3. Remove the pot from the heat and allow it to cool.

4. Once cooled, add in the alcohol and essential oils.

5. Transfer to a glass spray bottle for storage.

## How to Use

With either damp or dry hair, style your hair the way you want it, then spray the hairspray generously all over the hair to hold the style. If you want a stronger-hold hairspray, you can add more sugar.

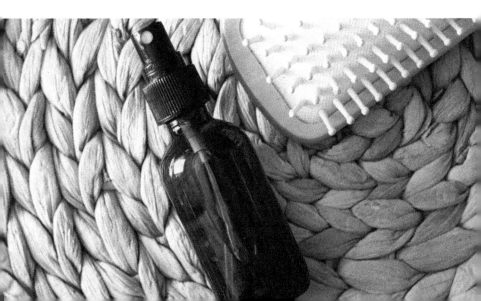

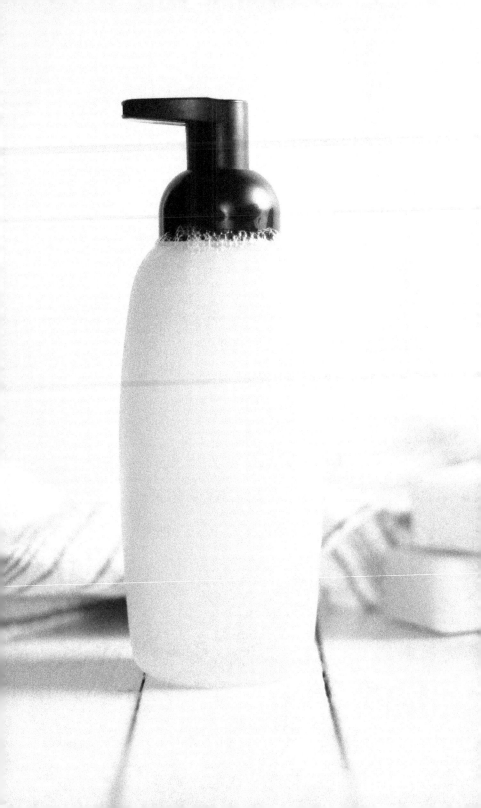

# Natural Shampoo

Traditional shampoos are made up of a lot of ingredients you will want to avoid. They have ingredients that have been known to mimic estrogen, which will cause hormone imbalances. They've also been known to contain carcinogens and ingredients that can also cause severe allergic reactions. Making your own with natural ingredients and essential oils is a much safer option. Plus, essential oils can be used for hair growth and strengthening.

After trying a few natural shampoos from the store, I decided to make my own because it is a whole lot cheaper! If you aren't a DIYer, you can most definitely find natural recipes that work great, but not without a price tag.

## Ingredients

- ¼ cup water (can substitute the water for coconut milk)
- ¼ cup castile soap
- ½ teaspoon jojoba oil (for dry hair, optional)
- 10–15 drops of essential oils (I have my favorite blends listed below)

## Instructions

1. Mix all the ingredients in a storage container. You can use an old shampoo bottle, foaming soap dispenser, or a mason jar.

2. After getting hair wet, apply a quarter-size amount to the hair and lather in. This shampoo is thinner than the typical shampoo, but it does lather up a ton! After shampooing, follow with an all-natural conditioner.

# Natural Shampoo Blends

## My Favorite Scent

6 drops wild orange essential oil
5 drops lime essential oil
4 drops bergamot essential oil
2 drops peppermint essential oil

## Blend for Hair Loss

6 drops rosemary essential oil
5 drops lavender essential oil
4 drops thyme essential oil
2 drops peppermint essential oil

## Best Scent for Men

6 drops lemongrass essential oil
4 drops sandalwood essential oil
4 drops melaleuca essential oil
2 drops bergamot essential oil

## Best Scent for Children

5 drops lavender essential oil
3 drops Roman chamomile essential oil
2 drops wild orange essential oil

# Natural Conditioner

I have the hair type that doesn't necessarily need conditioner. My hair is pin straight and extremely fine. I don't even need to brush it after showering, or ever.

My husband has the opposite thing going on. His hair is thick, coarse, and curly. And yes, all my kids got my hair. I was praying for one head of curls, but apparently, straight hair is dominant. He uses conditioner every time he showers and needs it to tame and moisturize his hair. This simple homemade conditioner has amazing benefits for your hair, and the best part: it is toxin-free.

I am using cocoa butter, coconut oil, jojoba oil, and aloe vera in this recipe. Cocoa butter is extremely moisturizing for the skin and works well at conditioning the hair. It provides shine, protects against split ends, and softens hair. Coconut oil has antibacterial properties, making it great for protecting the scalp against infections and lice. It is also effective for nourishing the hair and removing buildup.

Jojoba oil is often used as a natural remedy for dandruff because of its moisturizing properties. Using jojoba can also prevent hair loss and help thicken hair. If you have oily hair, you can eliminate this from the conditioner and try adding in a few drops of lemon instead. Aloe can reduce dandruff by repairing dead skin cells on the scalp and leave your hair fuller and shinier.

## Ingredients

+ 2 tablespoons cocoa butter
+ 2 tablespoons coconut oil
+ 1 tablespoon jojoba oil
+ 1 teaspoon aloe vera
+ 15–20 drops essential oil

## Instructions

1.  In a double boiler, melt the cocoa butter and coconut oil together. You can make your own double boiler by placing a glass bowl over a pot of boiling water.

2.  After the cocoa butter and coconut oil are melted together, remove from the heat. Let cool for 5 minutes, and then add in the jojoba oil, aloe vera, and essential oils.

3.  Stir well and pour into a storage container.

## How to Use

After washing hair with shampoo, add about a teaspoon of the conditioner to the scalp and massage in. Allow the mixture to sit on the hair for 2–3 minutes and then rinse out.

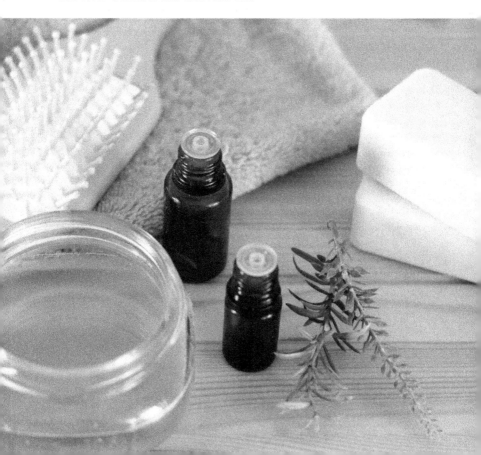

# Dry Shampoo

I washed my hair every day in high school; if I didn't, it would look greasy and oily. I always envied those people who could go several days without washing their hair, and it still looked good. My sister was one of those people. I assumed it was because we had different hair types. She has thick, coarse hair while, as I mentioned, I have thin and fine hair.

Once when I lamented this to her, she told me that you had to "train" your hair. Train your hair to not get greasy? Okay, whatever, I'll try it. Let me explain the basic science behind the "training." Your scalp produces oils; this is a good thing.

The oils help your hair to remain smooth and keep your hair from drying out and breaking off. When you wash your hair, you remove these oils, and your scalp produces more oils, so the more you wash, the more oils you're going to produce—catching on?

This same "training" has to happen when you are switching to natural shampoo and conditioners too. Just like anything else, your hair will need time to adjust. If your hair doesn't look perfect after the first time trying natural hair products, don't be alarmed. Be patient and trust the process. When I was "training," my dry shampoo was my best friend! When my hair looked greasy, I would use my dry shampoo to freshen it up. About a month in, my hair was used to the new schedule, and it adjusted nicely. I now only wash my hair twice a week, and it saves me a heck of a lot of time.

Mornings in my house can be chaotic; who can relate? I barely have time to brush my teeth, let alone shower. Once you have kids, going to the bathroom by yourself is a luxury. Dry shampoo has been my go-to probably more times than I should admit, but I promise I do shower.

Dry shampoo can allow you to preserve the natural oils in your hair and protect against dry scalp, all while saving you time. Dry shampoo absorbs the extra oils in your hair, making your hair look fresh and clean without shampooing. It usually comes in a spray or powder form.

**Dry Shampoo for Dark Hair**

- ✦ 3 tablespoons arrowroot powder
- ✦ 2–3 tablespoons cocoa powder
- ✦ 5 drops of essential oil of choice

**Dry Shampoo for Light Hair**

- ✦ ¼ cup arrowroot powder
- ✦ 1–2 teaspoon cocoa powder (you can omit this if you have very light or white hair)
- ✦ 5 drops of essential oil of choice

**Instructions**

Add arrowroot powder, cocoa powder, and essential oils to a bowl and mix well. Depending on the color of your hair will determine how much cocoa powder you will need. Start with less and add more until you reach the desired color. Transfer to an airtight container for storage.

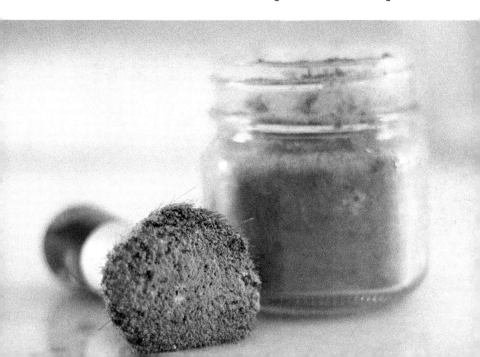

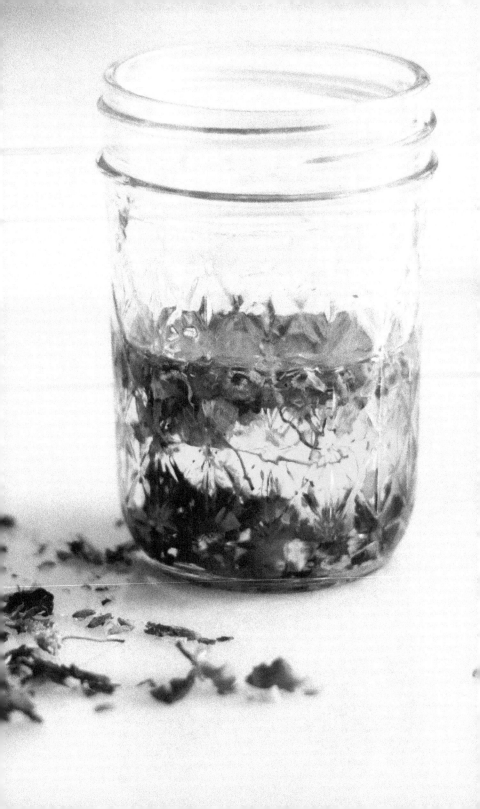

# Floral-Infused Body Balm

This floral-infused body balm smells as amazing as you can imagine, and it is so moisturizing to the skin. I am obsessed, to say the least. As the name suggests, it is made with floral-infused oil, giving it the best aroma and even more benefits for your skin.

It can be used on the hands or the body in place of regular lotion. I especially love to lather in this balm during the winter months when my skin is extra dry. It is made with simple, all-natural ingredients, making it perfect for sensitive skin. Even kids can use this one.

It will take four weeks to infuse your dried flowers into the oils, so you do have to do a little planning ahead for this one. Other than that, it is simple to make.

## How to Infuse Flowers Into a Carrier Oil

### Ingredients

+ Dried calendula
+ Dried lavender
+ Dried roses
+ Carrier oil

### Instructions

1. Add 2 tablespoons dried calendula, 1 tablespoon dried lavender, and 1 tablespoon of dried rose petals to ½ of a cup of carrier oil. I used ¼ cup coconut oil and ¼ cup grapeseed oil. Any carrier oil will do.

2. You will need to put it in a container with an airtight lid. I used a small mason jar. Place the mason jar in a cool, dark place for about 4 weeks.

3.   After the 4 weeks, strain the petals from the oil and use the floral-infused oil in the recipe.


## How to Make Body Balm

**Ingredients**

+   ½ cup mango butter
+   ½ cup floral-infused oil
+   10 drops wild orange essential oil

**Instructions**

1.   Melt the mango butter in a double boiler.

2.   Remove from heat and allow to cool slightly.

3.   Pour in floral-infused oil and wild orange essential oil.

4.   Stir until everything is well combined.

5.   Place the bowl in the refrigerator until it is set up. You want the mixture to be firm but not solid.

6.   Whip with a hand mixer until light and fluffy.

7.   Store in an airtight container.

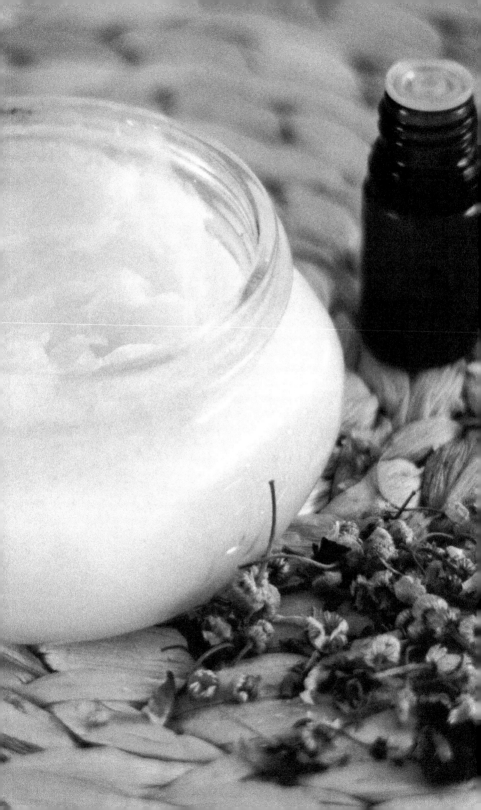

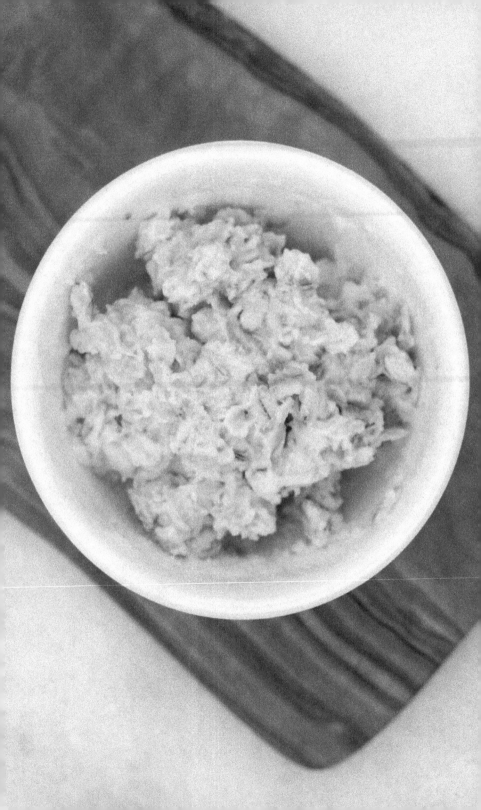

# Hand Mask for Dry, Cracked Skin

Whether your hands are dry from over-washing or cold weather, this hand mask can do wonders for your skin. It is made with avocado oil, beeswax, oatmeal, vitamin E oil, and lavender essential oil. All these ingredients can help to soothe and moisturize dry, cracked skin.

The recipe will make the perfect amount for one use. Apply it generously to the hands and massage it in well. The added-in oatmeal will help to exfoliate the skin and remove dead, dry skin cells.

For best results, put a pair of gloves on and leave the hand mask on overnight. In the morning, wash your hands clean with warm water. You can use this hand mask treatment a couple of times a week or as needed.

## Ingredients

+ 2 tablespoons avocado oil
+ 1 teaspoon beeswax
+ 2 tablespoons oatmeal
+ ¼ teaspoon vitamin E oil
+ 5 drops lavender essential oil

## Instructions

1. Place the avocado oil and beeswax in a double boiler and melt.

2. Remove from heat and add in remaining ingredients. Stir until everything is well combined.

3. Apply a generous amount to the hands. Rub them together to massage the lotion in and exfoliate the skin.

4. Leave on for at least 20 minutes and then wash off with warm water.

# Setting Spray

Setting spray can come in handy, especially on a hot summer day. This setting spray is made with all-natural ingredients to keep your makeup in place and from running. Making your own is much cheaper than buying it from the store, and it is much healthier for your skin.

I use a combination of vegetable glycerin, rosewater, witch hazel, and essential oils. The essential oils allow you to customize this spray just the way you like. My favorite essential oil to add is lavender because it is gentle enough for the face and has many benefits for the skin. Vegetable glycerin can help your makeup to stay in place for a longer period. Plus, it's super moisturizing for your skin and will give your makeup a pretty, glowing finish.

**Ingredients**

+ Spray bottle
+ 2 tablespoons vegetable glycerin
+ 2 tablespoons rosewater
+ 1 tablespoon of witch hazel
+ 3–5 drops lavender essential oil

**Instructions**

1. Pour all of the ingredients into a small spray bottle.

2. Secure lid and shake to make sure all the ingredients are well combined.

3. Mist the face lightly after putting on your makeup.

**Note**

Be sure to not use too much, or it can make your skin look oily.

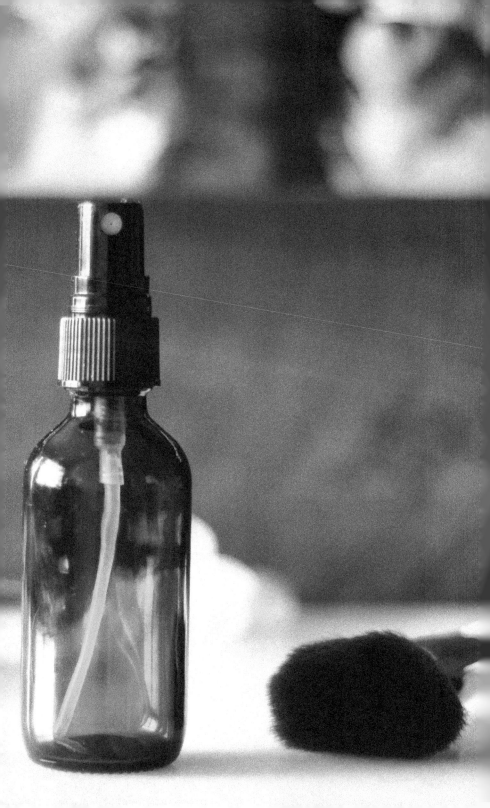

# Sugar and Soap Scrub Bars

We love making sugar scrub over here, and sometimes we get a little extra fancy and make sugar scrub bars. Sugar scrub bars are the perfect thing to exfoliate your skin. My favorite place to use these is on the face, hands, and feet.

For this recipe, we are going to use a soap base. You can make your own or purchase one. A soap base can be a solid or a liquid. I typically use a solid soap base that comes in a bar and melt it.

You will also need coconut oil for this recipe. The coconut oil will help to hold the sugar scrub together in the shape you decide to make, and it will add extra benefits for the skin. Coconut oil is moisturizing, can heal skin imperfections, and it can reduce inflammation.

And, of course, you can add in essential oils to customize your sugar scrub bar just the way you want.

**A Few of My Favorites**

**Lavender:** Soothing and calming
**Wild orange:** Uplifting and energizing
**Frankincense:** Anti-aging and skin-perfecting
**Bergamot:** Purifying and cleansing
**Roman chamomile:** Gentle and relaxing
**Peppermint:** Cooling and soothing

## Ingredients

+ ¼ cup coconut oil
+ ½ cup melted soap base
+ 1 cup of organic sugar
+ Silicone mold
+ Natural food coloring (optional)
+ 20–25 drops essential oils

## Instructions

1. In a small saucepan, melt your soap base. To make this faster, you can shred or cube the soap bar.

2. Add the coconut oil and sugar. Stir until well combined.

3. Mix in your food coloring if using and stir well.

4. Pour the mixture into your molds.

5. Allow the mixture to harden completely and then pop them out of the molds. This takes about 4 hours, depending on the size of the molds you are using.

6. You can store these in a glass mason jar or an airtight container.

## How to Use

Wet the skin where you plan to use the sugar scrub and then rub the bar onto the skin. Massage the sugar mixture into the skin to help exfoliate the skin. For best results, let it sit on the skin for a couple of minutes. Rinse off with warm water.

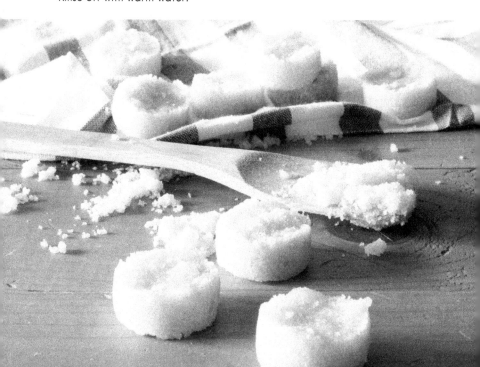

# Coffee Sugar Scrub

Believe it or not, coffee makes a great exfoliator for the skin. Pair it with sugar and essential oils, and it is the best natural skin care product. This coffee sugar scrub is a must during the cooler months when the skin is dry and flaky. It also makes the best gift for anyone or a great addition to the next girls' night.

You may not be surprised that the first ingredient on the list for a homemade coffee scrub is coffee grounds. It is best to use freshly ground beans, but any will do. Make sure you are using finely ground beans as more coarse grounds can be harsh on the skin.

Similar to the coffee grounds you use, the kind of sugar you use doesn't matter either. I prefer to use organic white sugar. You can use regular sugar or even brown sugar. Salt is great for exfoliating the skin too, but I find salt to work best on feet, elbows, and knees. Sugar is a safer option for the body, as it is softer.

My favorite essential oils to add to this coffee scrub are peppermint, lavender, and wild orange.

**Ingredients**

+ ½ cup coffee grounds
+ ½ cup sugar
+ ¼ cup coconut oil, melted
+ 10 drops peppermint essential oil

**Instructions**

1. Mix the dry ingredients in a small bowl.

2. Add in coconut oil, vanilla, and essential oils. Mix until well combined.

3. Scoop into a container with an airtight lid for storage.

**How to Use**

1.  Scoop out a generous amount and gently apply it to dry skin.

2.  Massage it using a circular motion and then allow it to soak into the skin for 5–10 minutes.

3.  Rinse off with warm water. Follow with a body moisturizer. For best results, use the coffee scrub up to three times a week.

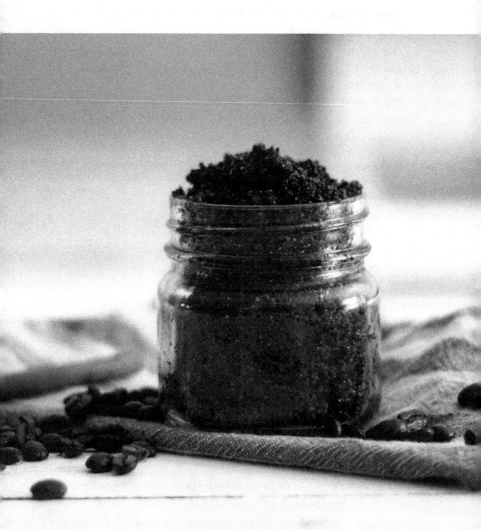

# Tinted Lip Balm

Every year, I make a batch of lip balm when the days get cooler and chapped lips become a problem. Sometimes, I get a little fancy and add a little color to it; my daughter especially loves when I do that. It makes the perfect all-natural lip color, and it makes your lips so soft.

Lip balm is simple to make and extremely cost-efficient. The recipe will make about twelve tubes of lip balm, lasting you all year long. You can buy empty lip balm containers or store these in any small, airtight container. The mixture will harden quickly, so it is important to work fast.

There are several natural powders you can use to make different color options. My favorite is hibiscus flower powder. Depending on how much you use, it makes a beautiful, rich pink color.

**Color Options**
**Pink:** Hibiscus flower powder
**Green:** Mica powder
**Red:** Beetroot powder
**Yellow:** Turmeric powder
**Brown:** Cocoa powder

You can lighten any color by adding a little arrowroot, or you can add cocoa powder to add warmth to your lip balm. You will only need a small pinch of powder to tint your lip balm. If you want to mix more than one powder, do that in a small bowl before adding it to your other ingredients to prevent it from clumping.

You can use several essential oils in your lip balm, depending on your preferred flavor and scent. Use mint essential oils for a cooling and soothing effect for chapped lips. If you use any citrus essential oils in your lip balm, be sure to keep it out of the sun. Citrus essential oils can cause a photo-toxic reaction, typically causing an exaggerated sunburn.

## Ingredients

+ 2 tablespoons beeswax
+ 2 tablespoons cocoa butter
+ 2 tablespoons coconut oil
+ ½ teaspoon of color of choice
+ 25 drops of essential oil
+ Lip balm tubes

## Instructions

1. Place all the ingredients (except essential oils and color) in a double boiler.

2. Melt all the ingredients together, stirring often.

3. Once all the ingredients are melted, remove from the heat, add your essential oils, powder color of choice, and mix well. Work fast, as the mixture will harden quickly after being removed from the heat.

4. With a small funnel, pipette, or old medicine dropper, fill the lip balm containers with the mixture.

5. Let tubes sit at room temperature for a few hours until cooled and completely hardened before capping them.

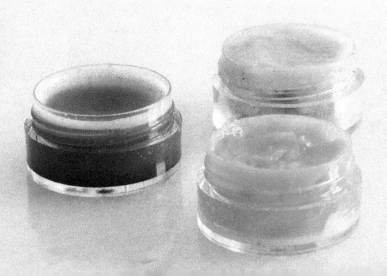

# Eyelash Serum

I am pretty plain Jane over here regarding style and fashion, but it doesn't take much exposure to the real world to know that long and thick lashes are in. If you need a little help in that area, don't worry. I have a natural solution for you.

Several essential oils can be used to strengthen and lengthen your hair. Making your own eyelash serum is easy and can be used to thicken and lengthen your lashes. All you need to make a serum are essential oils and carrier oil. The best carrier oil to use for this recipe is castor oil. Castor oil is great for hair growth. It is very moisturizing and can help to nourish hair follicles. Castor oil can thicken lashes within a few days of consistent use.

For this serum, we will use a combination of lavender, rosemary, and cedarwood essential oil. Lavender essential oil can produce more hair follicles to help thicken and strengthen hair. Rosemary essential oil is the top oil for hair growth and thickness. It helps to treat dry hair, as well as overly oily hair. Rosemary oil can also help prevent split ends. Cedarwood essential oil may promote hair growth and thickness and strengthen hair follicles.

Remember that we don't want to get essential oils in our eyes, so be careful when applying this eyelash serum. I find it easiest to apply this as you would mascara. I purchased a pack of empty mascara containers online that were inexpensive and made my serum in these.

### Ingredients

+ Lavender essential oil
+ Rosemary essential oil
+ Cedarwood essential oil
+ Empty mascara tube
+ Castor oil

## Instructions

1.  Add 10 drops of each essential oil to the mascara tube and top off with castor oil.

2.  It is best to apply this serum to the eyelashes once daily. I suggest applying at night time after washing your face and before bed. You can do it in the morning, but it may affect your eye makeup. Apply the serum daily for 6–8 weeks or as needed.

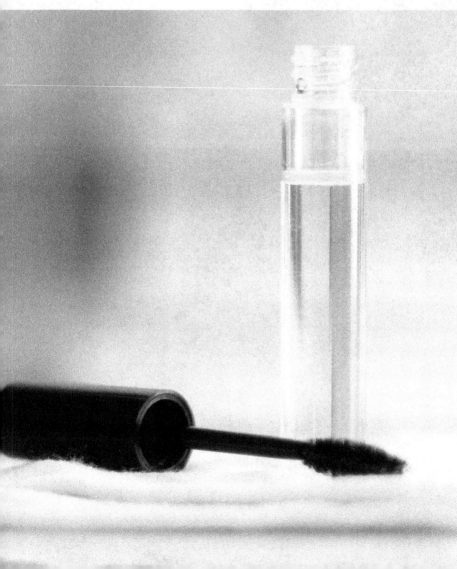

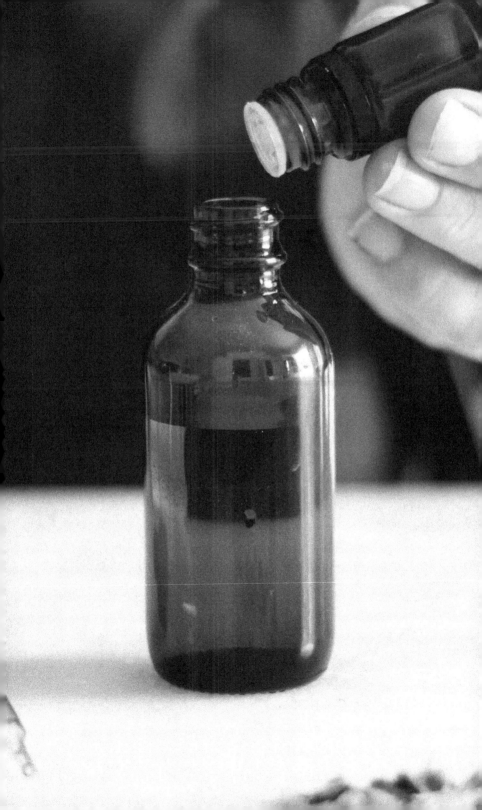

# Facial Serum

Making your own facial serum can be one of the best remedies for anti-aging. Several essential oils and carrier oils can reduce the appearance of wrinkles, fine lines, and aging spots.

At the end of the day, I am tired and just want to crawl into bed and skip my whole skincare routine. However, my face serum is one of those products I never miss putting on my face, even if it means I am putting it on a dirty, un-moisturized face. Not that I am suggesting doing this, but just being real.

Making your own serum is easy, cost-effective, and a great way to eliminate toxins going into your skin. Most conventional skincare products are loaded with ingredients we want to avoid putting on our skin and especially avoid putting on our face.

## Ingredients

+ 2 tablespoons jojoba oil
+ 3–5 drops of vitamin E oil (optional)
+ 5 drops sandalwood essential oil
+ 4 drops lavender essential oil
+ 3 drops frankincense essential oil

## Instructions

1. Add all the ingredients to a glass dropper bottle and tighten the lid.

2. Shake well before each use to make sure all ingredients are well combined.

3. Drop a small amount into the hand or directly onto the face and massage into the skin.

# Charcoal Face Mask

This face mask isn't your typical face mask. It is made with clay, coconut oil, activated charcoal, and essential oils. I know, I know; charcoal in a face mask? Yes, it will be messy and black, but it has many great benefits for your skin. It can help to cleanse, detox, purify, and can even help reduce acne and blackheads.

Activated charcoal is a fine black powder made from bone char, bamboo, wood, coconut husk, peat, petroleum pitch, coal, olive pits, or sawdust. You can make activated charcoal at home, or you can buy it. It will most likely be a one-time purchase, as it lasts forever, and you only need a little bit for each use.

Activated charcoal can be used to pull toxins and poisons out of the body. I bought some when we had a spider bite scare, and I decided I would always have some on hand, just in case.

**Ingredients**

+ 1 teaspoon bentonite clay
+ 1 teaspoon activated charcoal
+ 1 teaspoon coconut oil, melted
+ 2 drops of tea tree essential oil
+ Water, as needed

**Instructions**

1. Using a wooden spoon, mix the clay, charcoal, coconut oil, and tea tree essential oil in a small glass bowl. It is important to use glass and wood when working with clay.

2. If the mixture is too dry, you can add a little bit of water. Start with ⅛ of a teaspoon at a time until a creamy texture is reached.

## How to Use

1.  Wash face as usual, and then apply the charcoal mask.

2.  Spread evenly to whole face, avoiding eyes.

3.  Leave the mask on for 5–10 minutes. Rinse off with warm water. You may need to use a clean cloth to remove the mask.

4.  Follow up with an all-natural face moisturizer. (Psst, on next page.)

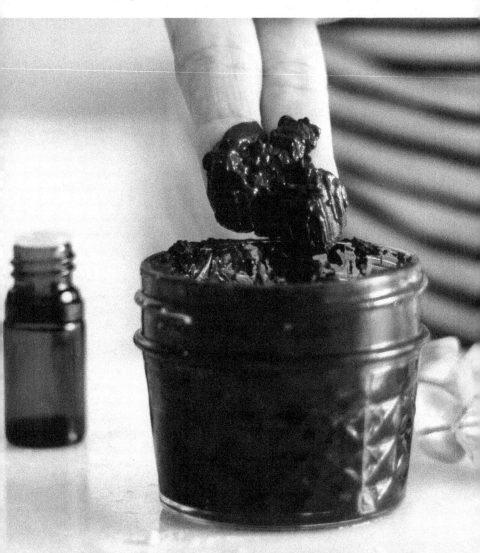

# All-Natural Face Moisturizer

The skin is the largest organ of the body, and everything you put on it gets absorbed into the bloodstream. So making my own lotions and moisturizers is important to me. I love that I can choose the best ingredients for my skin and know that they are all-natural. Making your own face moisturizer is easy and only requires a few ingredients.

The recipe calls for mango butter. You can replace the mango butter with shea butter or cocoa butter, depending on your skin type or preference. I find mango butter to be the least greasy of the three, and it has quickly become my favorite in almost all of my skincare recipes.

Similar to mango butter, the type of carrier oil you use is completely up to you. I am using fractionated coconut oil because it is light and moisturizing for the skin. You can also use jojoba oil, sweet almond oil, grapeseed oil, or reship oil. If you prefer, you can even use a combination of a few.

And of course, I add essential oils into this recipe. My favorites oils for the face are frankincense, rose, and lavender. All three of these oils have amazing benefits for anti-aging, skin blemishes, and skin tone. Plus, they give off the most beautiful floral aroma.

## Ingredients

+ ½ cup mango butter
+ 1 tablespoon fractionated coconut oil
+ ½ teaspoon vitamin E oil
+ 5 drops lavender
+ 5 drops frankincense
+ 5 drops rose

## Instructions

1. Place mango butter and coconut oil in a glass bowl.

2. Set the glass bowl over a pot of boiling water to create a double boiler. Melt the ingredients together.

3. Remove from heat; allow it to cool and set up.

4. Add in vitamin E oil and essential oils.

5. Whip it with a hand mixer to make it light and fluffy.

6. Store in an airtight container.

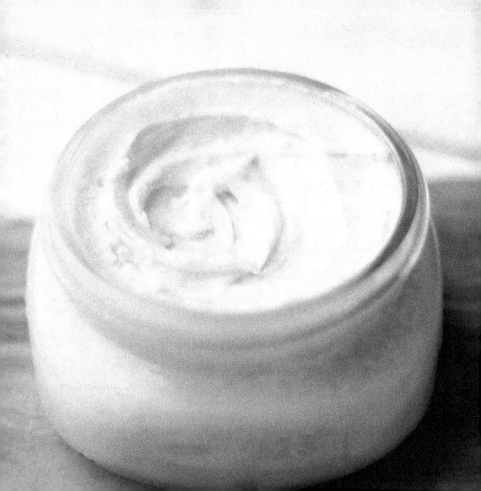

# Cooling Eye Masks

These cooling eye masks are the best addition to an at-home spa night or girls' day. Even though they are called eye masks, they are only meant to be used under the eye to help with puffiness and dark circles. All you need to make them are cucumbers, fresh mint leaves, aloe vera juice, lavender essential oil, and cotton rounds.

The fresh mint leaves and aloe vera juice are optional but make the masks more cooling and hydrating for the skin. You can leave out the mint altogether if you want, and you can use water instead of the aloe vera juice. Though, I highly recommend the aloe vera juice!

Aloe vera juice is a great source of antioxidants and vitamins that can hydrate the skin. It can reduce the appearance of fine lines and help with blemishes and breakouts. The fresh mint leaves give this eye mask a cooling and soothing effect. If making this for someone with sensitive skin, however, you may want to leave it out.

**Ingredients**

+ 1 cucumber, sliced
+ ¼ cup aloe vera juice
+ 3 fresh mint leaves (optional)
+ 3 drops of lavender essential oil (optional)
+ 10–15 cotton rounds, cut in half

**Instructions**

1. Place all the ingredients, except the cotton rounds, in a blender.

2. Blend until smooth.

3. Line a baking pan with wax paper.

4. Dip the cotton rounds into the cucumber mixture and place on the baking pan.

5. Place the pan in the freezer.

6. Once the cotton rounds are frozen, remove from pan and store in an airtight container.

**How to Use**

Remove two pieces of cotton rounds from the airtight container and place under the eyes. These are great to help you wake up in the morning or as an under-eye treatment before bed. For best results, use twice weekly.

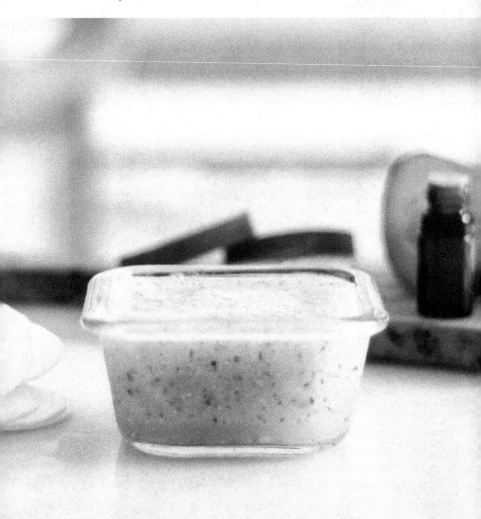

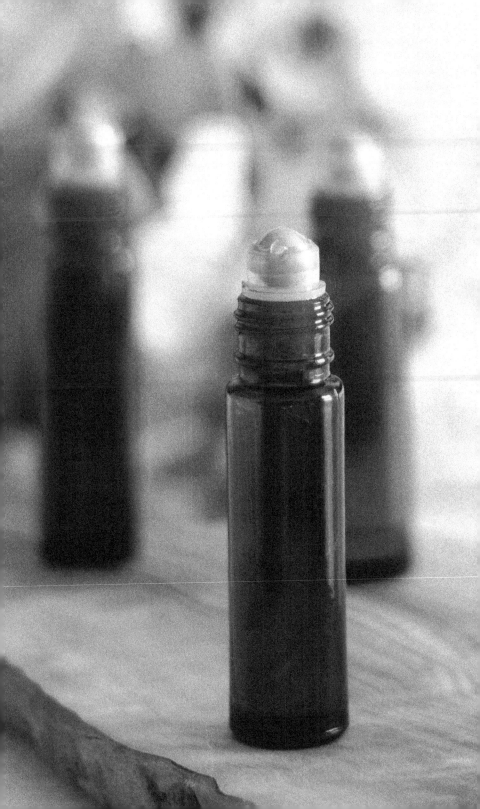

# CHAPTER 7

# Roller Bottle Recipes and Diffuser Blends

Roller bottles are the easiest way to apply essential oils topically and one of my favorite ways to use them. I keep them in my purse, all around the house, and in my car because you never know when you might need them.

To make a roller bottle, all you need are essential oils and a carrier oil. The type of oils you use will depend on the ailment you are dealing with. For an adult, it is best to use 15–30 drops of essential oils in a 10mL roller bottle and top it off with a carrier oil. For a child, it is recommended to use 5–10 drops of essential oil. Below are 20 different roller bottle recipes. Each recipe is based on using a 10mL roller bottle and diluted for an adult. You can adjust the drops of essential oils depending on for whom you are making it.

# Roller Bottle Recipes

## Clear Skin

8 drops lavender
8 drops tea tree
8 drops frankincense

Apply to the area of concern
as needed or until blemish
goes away.

## Immune Support

8 drops eucalyptus
6 drops wild orange
5 drops frankincense
4 drops clove

Apply to the bottom of feet,
down the spine, and/or on the
pulse points.

## Tummy Tamer

10 drops peppermint
10 drops ginger
5 drops wild orange
5 drops black pepper

Apply to the abdomen as needed.

## Respiratory Blend

8 drops eucalyptus
8 drops peppermint
6 drops lime
6 drops rosemary
4 drops thyme

Apply to the chest, upper back,
and on the bottom of the feet.

## Seasonal Threats

8 drops lemon
8 drops lavender
8 drops peppermint

Apply to the bridge of the nose
and chest several times a day.

## Head Tension

10 drops peppermint
8 drops lavender
8 drops frankincense

Apply to the temples and back of
the neck as needed.

## Ear Discomfort

8 drops tea tree
8 drops basil
8 drops lavender

Apply around the outside of the
ear canal 3–4 times daily until
discomfort goes away.

## Anti-Aging

5 drops frankincense
5 drops rose
3 drops helichrysum
2 drops myrrh
2 drops lavender

Apply to the area of concern
as needed.

## Dry Skin

10 drops myrrh
10 drops petitgrain
10 drops rose

Apply to the area of concern
as needed.

## Nail Care

10 drops lavender
10 drops myrrh
6 drops lemon

Apply on the nailbed twice daily
for best results.

## Calm and Relax

5 drops lavender
5 drops vetiver
4 drops cedarwood
4 drops frankincense

Apply to the pulse points
as needed.

## Joyful

6 drops wild orange
6 drops lime
6 drops bergamot
6 drops lemon

Apply to the pulse points
as needed.

## Focus

8 drops rosemary
8 drops peppermint
4 drops wild orange
4 drops frankincense

Apply to the pulse points
as needed.

## Positive Mood

8 drops bergamot
5 drops lime
5 drops lemon
5 drops lavender

Apply to the pulse points
as needed.

## Anti-Itch

6 drops basil
6 drops peppermint
6 drops tea tree
4 drops Roman chamomile
4 drops bergamot
4 drops eucalyptus

Apply to the area of concern
as needed.

## Bug Repellent

10 drops citronella

8 drops peppermint

4 drops cedarwood

4 drops lemon

4 drops lavender

Apply to exposed skin every 2 hours.

## Women's Perfume

8 drops bergamot

8 drops sandalwood

5 drops lavender

5 drops jasmine

Apply to the chest and wrists.

## Men's Cologne

10 drops bergamot

10 drops white fir

5 drops clove

5 drops lemongrass

Apply to chest and wrists.

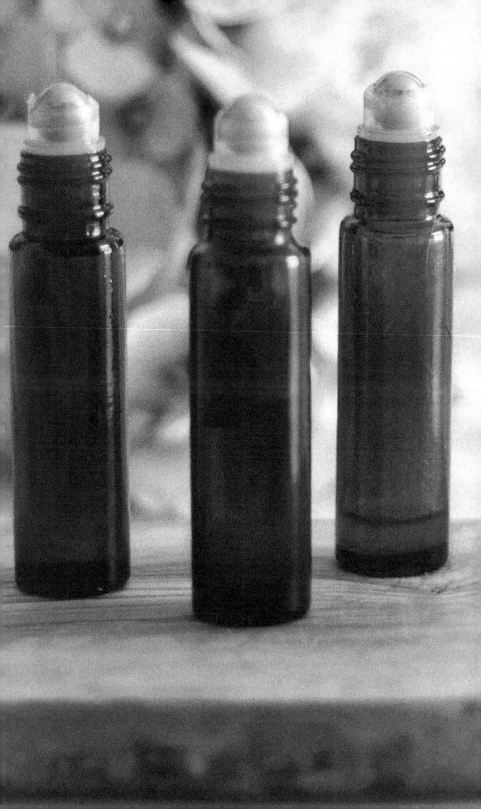

Diffusing essential oils is the most popular way to use essential oils. Not only do they make your house smell nice, but they also can benefit your body. When essential oils are diffused, you will receive aromatic benefits. Just by breathing in essential oils, they can affect your mood, boost your immune system, open up airways, or reduce stress.

Depending on the diffuser's size and the room you are diffusing in will determine how many drops of essential oils you will need to add to your diffuser. Typically, 4–6 drops is enough. Most diffusers will need to be filled with water before adding in your essential oils. If you prefer a stronger scent, you can always add more.

Below is a list of twenty different diffuser blends to try. I love trying new blends and diffusing them for the season. If you don't have every oil in a particular blend, that is okay. Just use what you have and get creative and come up with your own blends, too.

# Diffuser Blends

### Citrus

2 drops lemon
2 drops wild orange
2 drops lime

### Floral

2 drops lavender
2 drops magnolia
2 drops patchouli

### Woodsy

2 drops sandalwood
2 drops white fir
2 drops lemongrass

### Earthy

2 drops eucalyptus
2 drops frankincense
2 drops tea tree

### Relaxing and Calming

4 drops lavender
1 drop vetiver
1 drop frankincense

### Uplifting

4 drops lemon
1 drop spearmint
1 drop wild orange

### Energizing

2 drops peppermint
2 drops wild orange
2 drops lime

### Joyful

2 drops wild orange
2 drops lime
2 drops bergamot

### Positive Mood

2 drops bergamot
2 drops lemon
2 drops lavender

### Immune Support

2 drops frankincense
2 drops wild orange
2 drops clove

### Respiratory Relief

4 drops eucalyptus
1 drop peppermint
1 drop lime

### Focus Blend

2 drops rosemary
2 drops peppermint
2 drops wild orange

### Fresh and Clean

4 drops lemon
2 drops rosemary

### Stressed and Overwhelmed

3 drops lavender
2 drops copaiba
1 drop bergamot

### Rainy Day

4 drops lemon
2 drops vetiver
1 drop bergamot

### Cozy Night

3 drops eucalyptus
2 drops juniper berry
1 drop Siberian fir

### Fall

3 drops cinnamon bark
2 drops clove
1 drop cardamom

### Winter

2 drops Siberian fir
2 drops cinnamon
1 drop grapefruit
1 drop wintergreen

### Spring

2 drops juniper berry
2 drops grapefruit
2 drops lemon
1 drop cypress

### Summer

3 drops patchouli
3 drops wild orange
2 drops ylang-ylang

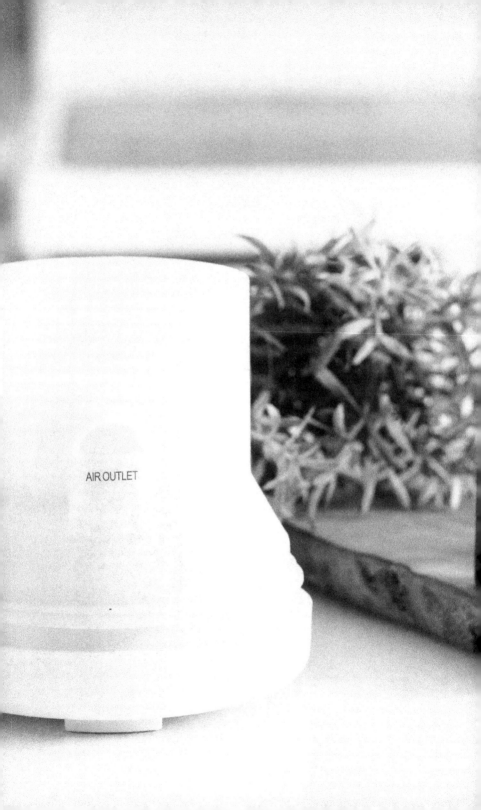

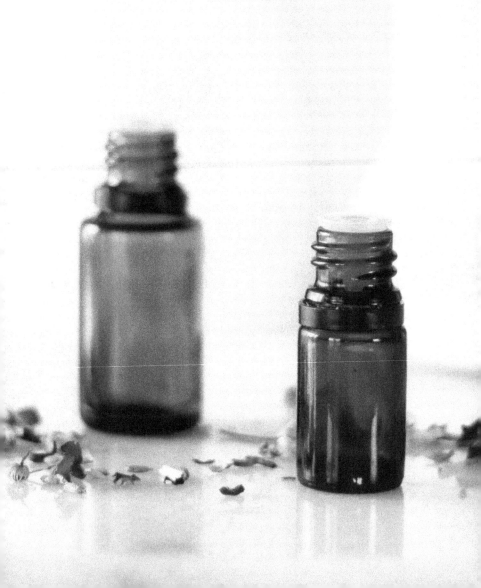

# Conclusion

I read a scary statistic about how many toxins the average human comes in contact with daily, which forever changed my life. I know I can't live a perfectly clean life or have full control of the air pollution around me, but I can do my best to provide a healthy home for my family. Sometimes I wish I didn't know as much as I do and could just trust that all the products sold are safe to use, but that isn't reality. I make a conscious decision about everything that I bring into my home, whether it be food, beauty products, or cleaners.

Bringing essential oils into my life has been such a game-changer for getting toxins out of my home and bringing natural solutions in. Feeling empowered to make your own cleaners, lotions, or candles is an awesome feeling and satisfying. Not only will these things come in handy for you and your family, but you will never run out of gift ideas again. Trust me; everyone loves getting homemade practical gifts that they can use.

I hope this book gave you an inspiration to "clean up" your home and start living a more simple, natural life. Making the change may seem hard at first, but once you get started, you will see how easy it is and how much money you can save. Getting toxins out of your home can be the first step in living a more holistic lifestyle. I hope you enjoyed this book and that it can be a reference for all of your essential oil questions and projects.

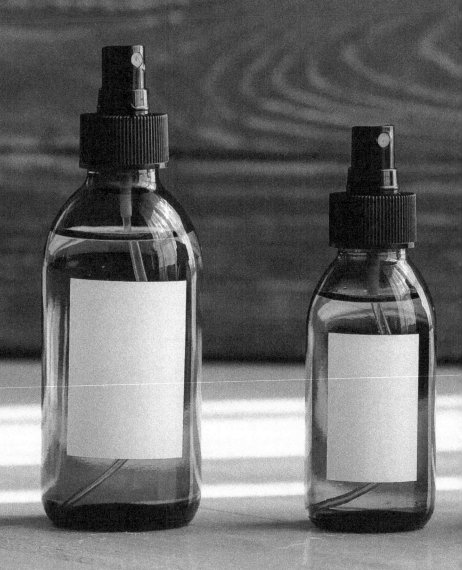

# Labels for Your Natural Products

# Chapter 1: Natural Kitchen Remedies

Lemon Tile Cleaner

Fruit And Veggie Wash

All-Purpose Spray

Beeswax Covers

Granite-Safe Spray

Homemade Wooden Spoon Butter

Liquid Dish Soap

Dishwasher Tablets

Stainless Steel Spray

Stainless Steel Polish

Oven Cleaner

Degreaser Spray

## Chapter 2: Natural Bathroom Remedies

Glass Cleaner

Bathroom Floor Scrub

Mold and Mildew Cleaner

Easy Homemade Toothpaste

Homemade Mouthwash

DIY Hand Sanitizer Spray

Reusable Cleaning Wipes

Tub and Sink Soft Scrub

Poo-Pourri Spray

## Chapter 3: Natural Laundry Remedies

Liquid Laundry Soap

Powder Laundry Soap

Fabric Softener

Spot Treatment

Fabric Softener

Natural Bleach

Dryer Sheets

Laundry Scent Boosters

Dryer Balls

## Chapter 4: Natural Bedroom Remedies

Linen Spray

Air Freshener

Furniture Polish

Massaging Lotion

Rosemary Mint Soy Candle

Roll-On Perfumes

# Chapter 5: Natural Baby and Kids Remedies

Diaper Cream

Baby Powder

Reusable Wipes and Spray Solution

Baby Wash

Baby Lotion

Natural VapoRub

## Chapter 6: Natural Bath and Beauty Remedies

Calming Bath Soak

Muscle Relaxing Bath Salts

Bedtime Tub Tea

Lemon Bath Bombs

Honey and Oatmeal Soap Bar

Natural Hair Spray

Natural Shampoo

Natural Conditioner

Dry Shampoo

Floral-Infused Body Balm

Charcoal Face Mask

Hand Mask for Dry, Cracked Skin

All-Natural Face Moisturizer

Setting Spray

Cooling Eye Masks

Sugar and Soap Scrub Bars

Coffee Sugar Scrub

Tinted Lip Balm
Eyelash Serum

Facial Serum

# Chapter 7: Roller Bottle Recipes and Diffuser Blends

# COOKING - BAKING
## conversions

### WEIGHT

| IMPERIAL | METRIC |
|----------|--------|
| 1/2 oz | 15 g |
| 1 oz | 29 g |
| 2 oz | 57 g |
| 3 oz | 85 g |
| 4 oz | 113 g |
| 5 oz | 141 g |
| 6 oz | 170 g |
| 8 oz | 227 g |
| 10 oz | 283 g |
| 12 oz | 340 g |
| 13 oz | 369 g |
| 14 oz | 397 g |
| 15 oz | 425 g |
| 1 lb | 453 g |

### MEASUREMENT

| CUP | ONCES | MILLILITERS | TBSP. |
|-----|-------|-------------|-------|
| 1/16 | 1/2 oz | 15 ml | 1 |
| 1/8 | 1 oz | 30 ml | 3 |
| 1/4 | 2 oz | 59 ml | 4 |
| 1/3 | 2.5 oz | 79 ml | 5.5 |
| 3/8 | 3 oz | 90 ml | 6 |
| 1/2 | 4 oz | 118 ml | 8 |
| 2/3 | 5 oz | 158 ml | 11 |
| 3/4 | 6 oz | 177 ml | 12 |
| 1 | 8 oz | 240 ml | 16 |
| 2 | 16 oz | 480 ml | 32 |
| 4 | 32 oz | 960 ml | 64 |
| 5 | 40 oz | 1180 ml | 80 |
| 6 | 48 oz | 1420 ml | 96 |
| 8 | 64 oz | 1895 ml | 128 |

### TEMPERATURE

| FAHRENHEIT | CELSIUS |
|------------|---------|
| 100 °F | 37 °C |
| 150 °F | 65 °C |
| 200 °F | 93 °C |
| 250 °F | 121 °C |
| 300 °F | 150 °C |
| 325 °F | 160 °C |
| 350 °F | 180 °C |
| 375 °F | 190 °C |
| 400 °F | 200 °C |
| 425 °F | 220 °C |
| 450 °F | 230 °C |
| 500 °F | 260 °C |
| 525 °F | 274 °C |
| 550 °F | 288 °C |

# About the Author

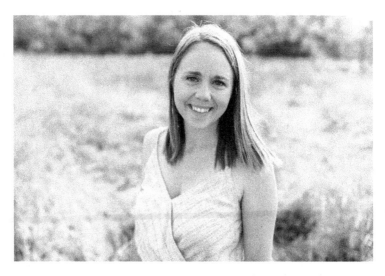

Laura Ascher is the creator and videographer of the blog and YouTube channel, *Our Oily House*. She lives in the Midwest with her husband Nathan and five kids. She started her blog in 2018 and enjoys sharing natural remedies and healthy recipes with her followers. You can find her online at ouroilyhouse.com or by searching "Our Oily House" on Facebook, YouTube, Instagram, or Pinterest.

Mango Publishing, established in 2014, publishes an eclectic list of books by diverse authors—both new and established voices—on topics ranging from business, personal growth, women's empowerment, LGBTQ studies, health, and spirituality to history, popular culture, time management, decluttering, lifestyle, mental wellness, aging, and sustainable living. We were recently named 2019 and 2020's #1 fastest growing independent publisher by *Publishers Weekly*. Our success is driven by our main goal, which is to publish high quality books that will entertain readers as well as make a positive difference in their lives.

Our readers are our most important resource; we value your input, suggestions, and ideas. We'd love to hear from you—after all, we are publishing books for you!

Please stay in touch with us and follow us at:

Facebook: Mango Publishing
Twitter: @MangoPublishing
Instagram: @MangoPublishing
LinkedIn: Mango Publishing
Pinterest: Mango Publishing
Newsletter: mangopublishinggroup.com/newsletter

Join us on Mango's journey to reinvent publishing, one book at a time.

Printed in the USA
CPSIA information can be obtained
at www.ICGtesting.com
JSHW012010140824
68134JS00023B/2354

9 781642 505481